HARVEY'S VIEWS ON THE USE OF
THE CIRCULATION OF THE BLOOD

COLUMBIA UNIVERSITY PRESS
SALES AGENTS

NEW YORK:
LEMCKE & BUECHNER
30–32 WEST 27TH STREET

LONDON:
HUMPHREY MILFORD
AMEN CORNER, E.C.

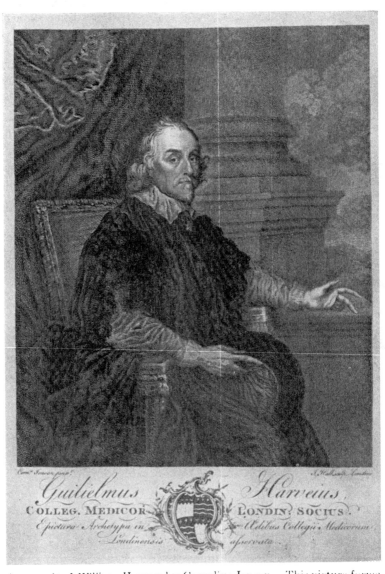

A portrait of William Harvey by Cornelius Jonson. This picture forms
the frontispiece of *Guilielmi Harveii Opera Omnia*, London, 1766.

HARVEY'S VIEWS ON THE USE
OF THE CIRCULATION
OF THE BLOOD

BY

JOHN G. CURTIS, M.D., LL.D.

FORMERLY PROFESSOR OF PHYSIOLOGY IN COLUMBIA UNIVERSITY
IN THE CITY OF NEW YORK

BASED ON A LECTURE DELIVERED IN 1907, BEFORE THE
JOHNS HOPKINS HOSPITAL HISTORICAL
CLUB AT BALTIMORE

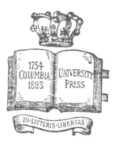

New York
COLUMBIA UNIVERSITY PRESS
1915

Set up and electrotyped.   Published December, 1915.

Norwood Press
J. S. Cushing Co. — Berwick & Smith Co.
Norwood, Mass., U.S.A.

PREFATORY NOTE

THE writings of William Harvey, as published by him, and the letters published as part of his works, are all in Latin. The passages from Harvey's works which appear in English in the present paper are in part translations by the late Dr. Willis, with changes, sometimes considerable, by the present writer. In large part, however, the translations from Harvey are not even based upon Dr. Willis's work, but have been made by the present writer directly from the original Latin. Naturally he assumes responsibility for whatever he prints in English to represent Harvey's words; and to attempt, in print, a more minute discrimination between his own work as a translator and that of Dr. Willis would be tedious and unprofitable. Whoever may wish to make such discrimination may readily do so, however, as, in the present paper, a reference is made by page and line in the case of each translated passage, not only to the Latin text of Harvey's *Opera Omnia*, published by the Royal College of Physicians of London in 1766, but also to Willis's English translation thereof, published by the Sydenham Society in 1847, and entitled "The Works of William Harvey, M.D." Such references to the Sydenham Society's edition are indispensable for another purpose, viz.: in order that to each translated passage from Harvey in the present

v

paper a context in English may readily be given by the reader.

It has seemed best that the various references to Harvey's Latin text should be made to that of the easily accessible *Opera Omnia* rather than to that of the rarer first editions of the several treatises. In the case of the passages quoted from the treatise *De Motu Cordis et Sanguinis in Animalibus* and from the treatise *De Generatione Animalium*, the Latin of the *Opera Omnia* has been collated by the present writer with that of the first editions. The first editions of the Exercises to Riolanus and of the various letters have not been accessible to him.

Much use has here been made of Harvey's private lecture notes, first published in 1886 by the Royal College of Physicians of London.

All the passages (except those from the Scriptures) quoted in the present paper from writers other than Harvey have been translated into English by the present writer directly from the original Greek text or the original Latin text, as the case may be.

JOHN G. CURTIS.

EDITORIAL NOTE

Professor Curtis, to whom I am indebted for much kindly help extended during a warm friendship of nearly thirty years, died September 20, 1913. One of his final requests was that his younger colleague arrange for the publication of the present paper, upon which its writer had been engaged for a period of several years and which happily was practically completed. This request, coming to me after the death of my friend, could be considered only as a command. It has, therefore, fallen to me to make a careful study of his text, to fill in with my own words occasional slight gaps, to make occasional verbal changes, to certify to the correctness of his numerous references, and to make the manuscript, written and in places rewritten many times with his own hand, ready for the press. This I have done with affection for his memory and with appreciation of his scholarly attainments. Dr. Curtis's work represents a more profound study of Harvey's ideas and comparison of them with those of the most important of Harvey's predecessors than has heretofore appeared. It is the work of one who from the background of the physiological science of to-day delighted in mastering the ideas of the fathers of modern physiology. If his work is to be summarized in a single sentence, it may be said that he has shown Harvey to be a disciple more of Aristotle than of Galen. Although Harvey had the courage and the originality to break away from him whose ideas had prevailed for fourteen centuries, and to find the truth in regard to the movement of the blood, he found much to approve in the master who had lived five hundred years before Galen. Harvey's true position in the world of physiological thought has not before been made known. Herein lies Professor Curtis's contribution to the history of his science.

FREDERIC S. LEE.

COLUMBIA UNIVERSITY,
June 1, 1915.

CONTENTS

CHAPTER I

HARVEY'S ATTITUDE TOWARD THE QUESTION OF THE USE OF

CHAPTER II

THE CIRCULATION AND THE FEEDING OF THE TISSUES .

CHAPTER III

RESPIRATION AND THE CIRCULATION

CHAPTER IV

THE CIRCULATION AND THE ARISTOTELIAN PRIMACY OF THE

CHAPTER V

PHYSICIANS *versus* PHILOSOPHERS — HARVEY FOR THE PHI-

CHAPTER VI

THE CIRCULATION AND THE PRIMACY OF THE BLOOD

ILLUSTRATIONS

HARVEY'S VIEWS ON THE USE
OF THE CIRCULATION
OF THE BLOOD

CHAPTER I

HARVEY'S ATTITUDE TOWARD THE QUESTION OF THE USE OF THE CIRCULATION

It is a happy moment for a physiologist when the train which is bearing him across the luxuriant plain of Venetia stops at the cry of "Padova!" If he have not informed himself too thoroughly about the sights which he will see at the Paduan University, he will enjoy his own surprise when he is ushered into the Anatomical Theater of Fabricius ab Aquapendente — a room in which standing-places rise steeply, tier above tier, entirely around a small central oval pit. Looking down into this, as he leans upon the rail, the traveler will realize with sudden pleasure that William Harvey, when a medical student, may often have leaned upon the self-same rail to see Fabricius demonstrate the anatomy of man. The place looks fit to have been a nursery of object-teachers, for it is too small to hold a pompous *cathedra;* and the veteran to whose Latin the young Englishman listened must have stood directly beside the dead body. To an American, musing there alone, the closing years of the sixteenth century, the

1

last years of Queen Elizabeth of England, which seem so remote to him when at home, are but as yesterday.

Recent, indeed, in the history of medicine is the year 1602, when Harvey received his doctor's degree at Padua and returned to London; but for all that we are right in feeling that our day is far removed from his. The tireless progress of modern times has swept on at the charging pace; but in Harvey's time books were still a living force which had been written in days five and six times as far removed from the student of Padua as he from us. Galen, the Greek who practised medicine at imperial Rome in the second century of the Christian era; Aristotle, who had been the tutor of Alexander the Great five hundred years before Galen, when Rome was but a petty state warring with her Italian neighbors; — these ancients were still great working authorities in Harvey's day.[1]

It is against this persistent glow of the Greek thought that Harvey stands out so vividly as the first great modern figure in physiology. But it rather heightens than lowers his achievement that it was by the ancient glow that he saw his way forward, admiring the past, but not dazzled by it. In his old age he bade a young student "goe to the fountain head and read Aristotle, Cicero, Avicenna"; and in talk with the same youth Harvey called the moderns by a name so roughly contemptuous that it will not bear repeating.[2] Yet in his old age, in the very act of extolling the ancients, he wrote as follows:[3] —

"But while we acquiesce in their discoveries, and believe, such is our sloth, that nothing further can be found out, the lively acuteness of our genius languishes and we put out the torch which they have handed on to us."

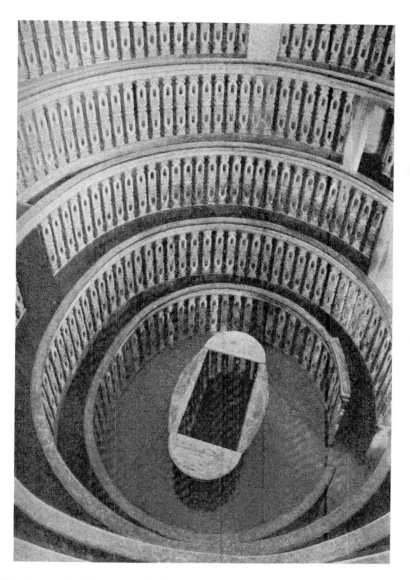

The Anatomical Theatre at Padua, where William Harvey listened to the
lectures of Fabricius ab Aquapendente.

It was in 1628, the year of his fiftieth birthday, that Harvey published, at Frankfort-on-the-Main, his famous Latin treatise entitled: "An Anatomical Exercise on the Motion of the Heart and Blood in Animals." A reader of to-day will be inclined to skim rapidly over the Introduction to this treatise and over much in the last three chapters; and probably he will take only a languid interest in the two brief Latin treatises which Harvey published in defense of the circulation, after more than twenty years of silence, in his seventy-first year, at Cambridge in 1649; these treatises being entitled: "Two Anatomical Exercises on the Circulation of the Blood, to Johannes Riolanus, Junior, of Paris."

The demonstration of the circulation in the treatise of 1628 is so irresistible that the ancient strongholds of belief crash to the ground at that summons like the walls of Jericho, and it seems a waste of time to scan the fragments. But for all that, the edifice which had stood for more than thirteen centuries was a goodly structure; and whoever shall have read Aristotle and Galen at first hand and shall then return to Harvey, will read with interest what the same reader treated as a mere foil for the great demonstration; and will realize that the irresistible quality of the latter is shared by Galen's demonstration that blood is naturally contained in the arteries.[4] Moreover, it will be seen that if the Greek of the second century could, like Harvey, appeal to observation and experiment, the English physician of the Renaissance, the student of Cambridge and Padua, was an apt pupil of the Greeks. Harvey could, and frequently and naturally did, view things from a Greek and ancient standpoint when proof of their

nature was unattainable.   This is to be seen not only in
his earlier and later exercises on the circulation, but also
in his last work, his "Exercise on the Generation of
Animals" with appended essays, published in Latin at
London in 1652, in Harvey's seventy-third year, two
years after the appearance of the exercises addressed
to Riolanus.   This treatise On Generation deals also at
various points with the blood and the circulation, as do
in addition Harvey's published Latin letters.   We shall
find, too, the same leaning upon the ancients as immediate precursors in thinking, if we turn back from
the publications of Harvey's old age to the very first
written words of his which we possess, private lecture
notes jotted down by him in his thirty-seventh year
for use in 1616 — notes happily printed and published in 1886.[1]   In these notes, written more than
eleven years before the publication of his most famous
treatise, he sets forth for the first time, though briefly,
the circulation of the blood, that physiological truth
which to my mind is completely and indisputably
Harvey's own discovery.   It is with Harvey as the
interpreter, not the maker, of this discovery, that I
shall venture to deal in this paper.

In his old age the great discoverer recorded his own
attitude, as an interpreter, in the following words : —

"That freedom which I freely concede to others, I demand with
good right for myself also ; liberty, that is, in dealing with obscure
matters, to bring forward, to represent, the truth, that which seems
probable, until the falsity thereof shall clearly be established." [1]

In 1636, eight years after he had published the treatise
which now seems so convincing, Harvey was in Nurem-

berg and wrote to Caspar Hofmann, M.D., a professor of repute who lived there, offering to demonstrate the circulation to him. In his letter Harvey quotes impatient words of his German colleague, which show that in the face of proof the circulation still seemed to some men of high standing too useless to be true. Harvey says to Hofmann : —

"You have been pleased to reproach me rhetorically and chastise me tacitly as one who seems to you 'to accuse and condemn nature of folly as well as error, and to impose the character of a most stupid and lazy craftsman on her, since he would permit the blood to relapse into rawness and to return repeatedly to the heart to be concocted again ; and, as often, to the body at large to become raw again ; and would permit nature to ruin the made and perfected blood in order that she may have something to do.' " [6]

To this attack Harvey calmly rejoins as follows, speaking of the blood : —

"As to its concoction and the causes of this its motion and circulation, especially their final cause, I have said nothing, indeed have put the subject by entirely and deliberately ; as you will find set down in plain words and otherwise if you will be pleased to read again chapters VIII and IX." [7]

More than twelve years later still, in defending the circulation against Riolanus, Harvey finds it necessary to say : —

"Those who repudiate the circulation because they see neither the efficient nor the final cause of it, and who exclaim ' Cui bono ? ' — (As to which I have brought forward nothing so far ; it remains to be shown) — plainly ought to inquire as to its existence before inquiring why it exists ; for from the facts which meet us in the circulation regarded as existing, its uses and objects are to be sought." [8]

In spite, however, of these disclaimers of formal position Harvey had repeatedly intimated, by the way, what was crossing his mind as to the meaning of the circulation, to set forth the proofs of which had been his main concern. Even in the eighth chapter to which Harvey appealed in support of his disclaimer Hofmann could have pointed to two passages as affording from his standpoint a basis for his attack. In the second and shorter of these two passages Harvey says of a vein as compared with an artery : —

"This is a way from the heart, that to the heart; that contains cruder blood, effete and rendered unfit for nutrition; this, concocted, perfect, alimentary blood." [9]

Harvey, indeed, as we shall find abundant evidence, was both an observer and a speculator. In the latter rôle he was not far removed from his physiological predecessors of two thousand years; as an observer it was his great merit to lead the physiologists of his time and to point out to those of all later centuries the path which they must follow.

CHAPTER II

THAT Harvey frequently took refuge in speculation need excite no surprise. In the seventeenth century, even with his extraordinary contributions of observed fact to the knowledge of the circulation of the blood, the paucity of physiological knowledge in general and of experimental methods was so great that at every turn a thinking man was tempted to fill in the gaps with that which was beyond his powers of ocular demonstration. Contemplation of the circulation, indeed, led Harvey into contemplation of widely diverse problems of the life process. The feeding of the tissues, the significance of respiration, the cause of the heart-beat, the relative importance of the heart and the blood in the bodily hierarchy, the bodily heat and its source, and the seat of the soul — to these and other topics he gave much attention, and these we must consider. Let us begin with the circulation and its relation to the feeding of the tissues.

In the chapter of Harvey's book which follows at once upon the brief qualitative statement quoted at the end of our last chapter, Harvey himself brings us face to face with the difficult quantitative question raised by his triumphant proof of the circulation. He says : —

7

"The blood under the influence of the arterial pulse enters and is impelled in a continuous, equable, and incessant stream into every part and member of the body, in much larger quantity than were sufficient for nutrition or than the whole mass of fluids could supply." [10]

Here we see that the rapid renewal of the blood in "every part and member of the body" presented itself to Harvey's own mind as calling for some other explanation than the simple feeding of the tissues. The question of "cui bono" which his discovery raised is still but incompletely answered; in Harvey's day it was almost unanswerable. In dealing from time to time with its main features he himself, as we shall see, could only bring forward inadequate observations and shift his ground from one erroneous doctrine to another. In justice to his opponents, who seem to us so unreasonable, let us remember how prodigious this new question of "cui bono" must have seemed when the circulation itself was a novelty. Let us remember also that for nearly two thousand years the tissues had been held to feed themselves tranquilly out of the contents of the vessels in a way fitly expressed by the old simile of irrigation ditches in a garden — a simile which Aristotle and Galen had borrowed in turn from Plato. [11]

But if Harvey saw only too well that the feeding of the tissues could not explain the circulation, he had at least seen plainly how the doctrine of the circulation clarified the ancient but current doctrine as to the absorption of the digested food. The portal vein had been accepted as the route of this absorption. No doubt both Aristotle and Galen had seen its ruddy contents; at any rate both had concluded that the chyle was changed within the portal vein into a crude approximation to blood.[12]   That the same vessel should carry to the liver altered chyle, and from the liver blood to nourish the stomach and intestines, had involved a difficulty which Galen had met with characteristic cleverness.   He had cited in support of such a reversal of flow the flow of the bile into the gall-bladder and out by the same duct, the movement of food and vomit into and out of the stomach by the œsophagus, and the relation of the os uteri to impregnation and parturition.[13] Harvey says : —

"For the blood entering the mesentery by the cœliac artery and the superior and inferior mesenterics proceeds to the intestines, from which along with the chyle that has been attracted into the veins it returns by their numerous ramifications into the vena portæ of the liver, and from this into the vena cava, and this in such wise that the blood in these veins has the same colour and consistency as in other veins, in opposition to what many believe to be the fact. Nor need we hold the improbable belief that two inconveniently opposed movements take place in the whole capillary ramification, namely, movement of the chyle upward, of the blood downward. Is not the thing rather arranged as it is by the consummate providence of nature?   For were the chyle mingled with the blood, the crude with the concocted in equal proportions, the result would not be concoction, transmutation, and sanguification, but rather, because they are reciprocally active and passive, a mixture, their union with one another producing something intermediate, precisely as when wine is mixed with water and [in] vinegar and water [oxicratum].   But when a minute quantity of chyle is mingled with a large quantity of blood flowing by, a quantity of chyle that bears no notable proportion to the blood, the effect is the same, as Aristotle says, as when a drop of water is added to a cask of wine, or the contrary; the resulting total is not a mixture, but is either wine or water.   So in the dissected mesenteric veins we do not find chyme or chyle and blood, separate or mingled, but only blood, sensibly the same in color and consistency as in the rest of the veins." [14]

In a second passage of the same chapter,[15] Harvey returns to this subject; and again, twenty-one years later, in his first exercise to Riolanus, as follows: —

"Our learned author mentions a certain tract of his on the Circulation of the Blood: I wish I could obtain a sight of it; perhaps I might retract. But had the learned writer been so disposed, I do not see but that, having admitted the circular motion of the blood (and in the veins, as he says in the eighth chapter of the third book,[16] the blood incessantly and naturally ascends, or flows back, to the heart, as in all the arteries it descends or departs from the heart), all the difficulties which were formerly felt in connection with the distribution of chyle and the blood by the same channels are brought to an equally satisfactory solution; for all the mooted difficulties vanish when we cease to suppose two contrary motions at once in the same vessels, and admit but one and the same continuous motion in the mesenteric vessels from the intestines to the liver." [17]

From this passage we see, in passing, that Harvey at the age of seventy made little account of Caspar Aselli's discovery of the lacteals, published twenty-two years before in 1627,[18] the year before the announcement of the discovery of the circulation. Harvey's mind was focused on the blood, its motion and its meaning; this was to him the subject of prime importance. The ancient doctrine of the feeding of the tissues provided an insufficient reason for the existence of what his observations and his experiments revealed to him.

CHAPTER III

RESPIRATION AND THE CIRCULATION

So the feeding of the tissues could not sufficiently account, to Harvey's mind, for the swiftness of the circulation. What could? It is easy for us to recite the multitudinous modern duties of the blood as a bearer of cells and of chemicals from point to point and as a protector against poisoning; above all it is easy to exclaim "respiration"; — to read the most striking part of the riddle by knowing the answer which was wrung laboriously from Nature after Harvey had died. It is easy for us to see that speedy death from loss of the circulating blood is practically the same as death from ligature of the arteries of the brain, or from drowning, or strangulation, or a broken neck. But this was veiled from him, and what best accounts for the volume and swiftness of the Harveian circulation was, in Harvey's day, a stumbling block to its acceptance; for no adequate reason was apparent why the whole mass of the blood should traverse the lungs, or why, if the veins receive their blood from the arteries, the venous blood should differ in color from the arterial.

Let us remember that throughout Harvey's life air was still an elementary body in the eyes of many and, for all, blood was a quite mysterious, ruddy, hot, vital liquid. Only weak magnifying glasses were available for him, and the powerful lenses of Malpighi and van Leeuwenhoek had not yet revealed to the world either

11

capillary or blood-corpuscle. Moreover, the gossiping John Aubrey, the man who had been advised about his youthful studies by Harvey, wrote of him some years after his death, that "he did not care for Chymistrey, and was wont to speake against them [the chemists] with an undervalue."[19] Where would physiology be to-day, had not histology and chemistry long stood in the forefront beside her?

In a passage of the treatise of 1628 Harvey speaks of respiration, as follows : —

"And now it has come to this, that it would seem better worth while and more straightforward for those who seek the path by which in man the blood passes through the vena cava into the left ventricle and the venous artery,[20] to be willing to search for the truth by dissecting animals, in order to look for the reason why in the larger and more perfect animals, when full grown, nature chooses to make the blood percolate through the parenchyma of the lungs rather than take wide open paths as in all other animals (it being understood that no other path and transit can be thought out) : — whether it is because the larger and more perfect animals are hotter and when they are full grown their heat is more ignited, so to speak, and prone to be smothered, that there is this permeation and transfer through the lungs in order that the heat may be tempered by the inspired air and guarded from boiling up and smothering — or for some other similar reason. But to determine these matters and explain them completely were to enter on a speculation as to the purpose for which the lungs are made. About these and their use and motion, and the whole subject of ventilation and the need and use of air, and other matters of this sort, and about the various different organs created in animals by reason thereof, although I have made a vast number of observations, I shall not speak till I can more conveniently set them forth in a treatise apart, lest by wandering at this point too far from my subject, which is the motion and use of the heart, I should seem to deal with something else and leave my position, to confuse and evade the question." [21]

Farther on in the same treatise Harvey says : —

"Moreover, the reason why the lungs have vessels so ample, both vein and artery, that the trunk of the venous artery exceeds in size the crural and jugular branches taken both together; and the reason why the lungs are so full of blood as we know them to be by experience and inspection (heeding Aristotle's warning,[22] and not deceived by the inspection of such lungs as we have removed from dissected animals from which all the blood had flowed out) — the reason is, that in the lungs and heart is the storehouse, the source, the treasury of the blood, the workshop of its perfection."[23]

So the great Englishman gropes for a moment or two by the light of ancient Greek doctrines and puts the question of respiration by. But this very attitude shows Harvey's thought to be in such contrast with the thought of to-day that in order to understand him we need to learn more fully his views of respiration; and we find with satisfaction that in his lecture notes of more than eleven years before he had not put this question by, for he had been called upon to lecture upon the uses of the lungs. We must seek in his lecture notes, therefore, for what he had thought those uses to be. These notes, however, we shall be unable to follow unless now, first of all, we shall give the floor for a while to the ancients; for from their doctrines Harvey necessarily took his cue, like the other thinkers of his time.

The momentous physiological facts that the living body of man, beast, or bird, is warm of itself and that its cooling means its death, must always have struck and impressed the human mind, whether trained or untrained. More than nineteen centuries before Harvey certain thoughts of Aristotle were recorded as follows : —

"In animals all the parts and the entire body possess a certain innate natural heat; wherefore they are sensibly warm when living, the reverse when making an end and parting with life. In the animals which have blood the origin of this heat is necessarily in the heart, in the bloodless kinds in the analogue thereof; for all work up and concoct the nourishment by means of the natural heat, the master part most of all. Life persists, therefore, when the other parts are chilled; but if what resides in this one be so affected total destruction ensues, because upon this part they all depend as the source of their heat, the soul being as it were afire within this part; that is, within the heart in the animals which have blood, in the bloodless kinds in the analogue thereof. Necessarily, therefore, the existence of life is coupled with the preservation of the heat aforesaid, and what is called death is the destruction thereof." [24]

This heat which is innate in all living animals was styled by Aristotle not only "innate" but "natural," "vital,"[25] and "physical,"[26] it being indispensable to life and to the working of the soul. He held the continued existence of the innate heat to depend upon conditions similar to those under which a fire is kept alive, viz.: protection both from burning out and from extinction due to external forces. Yet the true nature of combustion was not settled till more than a century after Harvey's death. The fact that air is necessary to fire must always have been a matter of common knowledge. Therefore, the views of the relations of air to fire maintained by Aristotle nearly twenty-one centuries before the discovery of oxygen did not seem naïve to Harvey, whatever they may seem to us. Aristotle held that air exerts upon fire a cooling influence which saves it from burning out too fast; and that the same influence is exerted upon the vital innate heat of animals by the air which they breathe in, or the water which bathes their gills.[27] Moreover, Aristotle says : —

"Why those animals breathe most which have lungs containing blood, is plain from this : that the warmer an animal is, the greater need it has of cooling, while at the same time the breath passes easily toward the source of warmth within the heart. But the way in which the heart is pierced through toward the lung must be studied from dissections and from the history of animals which I have written. In general terms, then, it is the nature of animals to need cooling on account of the firing of the soul within the heart." [28]

In the treatise styled the "History of Animals," to which he refers us, Aristotle says : —

"There are also channels from the heart which lead into the lung and divide in the same way as the windpipe, and they accompany the channels from the windpipe throughout the entire lung. The channels from the heart lie uppermost ; but no common channel exists, for it is by contact [29] that they receive the breath and transmit it to the heart." [30]

The collection of ancient Greek commonly called the "Works of Hippocrates" is judged to be of the fifth and fourth centuries B.C. There is included in this collection a brief treatise on the heart ; and in this occurs the earliest known account of the structure and use of the semilunar valves, which together with the rest of the cardiac valves were unknown to Aristotle. In the same Hippocratic treatise the doctrine is adhered to of the entrance of air into the heart for cooling purposes, both the right and the left ventricle being specified as receiving it. The author says : —

"The vessel which leads out of the right ventricle . . . closes toward the heart, but closes imperfectly, in order that air may enter, though not very much." [31]

This piece of incorrect physiology may well have received support from the fact that the pulmonary semilunar valve is commonly found to be not quite competent when the dead and dissected pulmonary artery of the bullock is distended with water — an observation which the ancient author intimates that he has made,[32] though he does not specify the creature dissected.

Nearly five hundred years after the death of Aristotle, the analogy between life and flame was discussed, formally and at some length, by Galen. He knew his Aristotle well, and agreed with him as to the importance of respiratory cooling for protracting the indispensable heat of animals.[33] But we find Galen dealing with the uses of respiration in a less simple way than Aristotle. In a polemical treatise Galen debates the question whether "the breath drawn in in respiration" actually enters the heart, or whether it cools it without entering it. He says: —

"It is possible that the whole is breathed out again, as was believed by most physicians and philosophers, and those the keenest, who say that the heart, while it craves to be cooled, is in need not of the substance, but of the quality [34] of the breath, and that the use of respiration is indicated by the part. . . . I have shown in my treatise on the use of respiration that either an absolutely minute quantity, or none at all, of the substance of the air, is taken into the heart." [35]

It is clear, however, that Galen, when delivering himself of the foregoing, was a trifle carried away by the ardor of contention; for in the very treatise to which he refers us, as well as elsewhere, he not only dilates upon the cooling effects of breathing, but admits the entrance of air into the heart for a definite physiological purpose. This purpose, however, which we shall study later, is not cooling and is counted of secondary importance by Galen. Nevertheless, he goes so far as to say this : —

"That some portion of the air is drawn into the heart in its diastole and fills the vacuum which is produced, is sufficiently shown by the very magnitude of the dilation." [36]

In his treatise "On the Use of the Parts of the Human Body" Galen takes a more judicial tone in the following brief, calm summary : —

"The use of the respiration of animals arises from the heart, as has been shown. The heart itself needs in some sort the substance of the air; but, first and foremost, it craves to be cooled, because it boils with heat. The heart is cooled by the cool quality of inspiration; but expiration also cools, by pouring out that which seethes within the heart and is, in a way, burned up and sooty." [37]

Thus do we see the modern products of respiration foreshadowed.

Galen believed that the heat of animals is safeguarded also by the entrance of cooling air through the pores of the skin into the arterial system, and by the exit through these pores of injurious fumes out of the arteries.[38]   In the introduction to Harvey's great treatise of 1628 [39] the English physician riddles with adverse arguments this doctrine of Galen; to this we shall return later, as we shall to Galen's belief that the brain draws cooling air directly into its ventricles out of the nares through the cribriform plate of the ethmoid bone.[40]

In passing from Aristotle to Galen we have crossed nearly five centuries.   Now let us pass at a leap across fourteen centuries more, from Galen at imperial Rome under Septimius Severus to Harvey at London under King James the First.   Having briefly scanned the doctrines of the Greeks, let us take up our study of respiration in Harvey's private lecture notes of 1616.   His crabbed handwriting has been deciphered by experts, and his notes have been both photographed and printed. If we seek therein for his thoughts about respiration, and track them through the jungle of abbreviated careless Latin and racy English in which they were jotted down, we shall find them Galenic in part, but also denying a truth which Galen had accepted.   Harvey's notes are often too disconnected for quotation, calling rather for paraphrase or summary;   and to make either is a task which one cannot approach without diffidence, especially as this task involves translation also.   Of what I have ventured to prepare to represent parts of Harvey's note-book in the present paper some passages are simple translations, such English words as Harvey interspersed being transcribed.   Naturally such passages are included between quotation marks.   These are not used, however, in the case of a paraphrase or summary, even if it contains scattered English words which are Harvey's own.

Harvey fully shared the ancient view of the supreme importance of the heat of animals.   In his note-book he, like Galen, deals with respiration under the heads: first, of a possible absorption of some of the substance of the air;   and, second, of cooling and ventilation. Let us first take up the second head.   Harvey says : —

"Without nourishment life cannot be, nor nourishment without concoction, nor concoction without heat, nor heat without ventilation;" for heat perishes either of wasting or of smothering; "so there is cooling and ventilation of the native heat, ventilation especially." [41]

His words contain reminders of Aristotle; [24] and he continues about respiration in a vein as ancient as Hippocrates, [42] as follows : —

"Nothing is so necessary, neither sense nor food. Life and respiration are convertible terms, for there is no life without breathing and no breathing without life. If the eye be cut out there is an end of seeing; if the legs be cut off there is an end of walking; if the tongue, of speech, et cetera; if respiration, there is an end of everything immediately." [43]

When Harvey jotted this down he had in mind a Galenic passage which doubtless had become the common property of all physicians in his day; for the removal of eye and legs figures in the first chapter of Galen "On the Use of Respiration." [44] Harvey continues : —

"Hence large animals are much warmer and breathe frequently, because they have need of greater cooling and ventilation inasmuch as they very greatly abound in blood and heat." [45]

In the margin opposite this passage there is written : —

"Why and how air is needed by animals which breathe and also air is necessary to a candle and to fire see W. H."

We may conjecture that this note refers to Harvey's promised treatise on respiration, which was never published.

So far Harvey has simply reiterated the ancient doctrine of cooling and ventilation, as in the passages quoted previously from the treatise of 1628. We shall find it very interesting to see how he deals with the other ancient doctrine that some of the substance of the air joins the blood in respiration. That this is true, gas analysis and the mercurial air-pump have taught us; but in this matter modern demonstration does but confirm, extend, and make precise one of the oldest of physiological beliefs. Regarding this we must now give the floor once again to the ancients, in order to make Harvey comprehensible.

Even in the days of Empedocles and Hippocrates, in the fifth and fourth centuries before Christ, men wrote of something derived from the outer air being present, for the use of the organism, in the vessels which also contain the blood.[46] To express this derivative of the outer air the ancient Greeks employed the word "*pneuma*" (πνεῦμα), the fundamental meaning of which seems to have been "air in motion." Various meanings were acquired by "*pneuma*," such as the breath of living things, the wind, or simply the air, or what we mean by the words "gas," "vapor," "steam," "exhalation," "emanation." The Latin word equivalent to "*pneuma*" is "*spiritus*," and so the English derivative of this, the word "spirits," came into use to express various meanings of the Greek "*pneuma*." A Hippocratic writer tells us that "the spirits cannot stand still, but go up and down" in the blood vessels. The word "spirits" here designates a derivative of the outer air crudely mingled with the blood.[47] To this writer the distinction between veins and arteries was unknown.

In the genuine works of Aristotle this Hippocratic

doctrine does not reappear, though it is fairly certain that Hippocratic treatises which contain it were written before Aristotle's time. We have seen that the entrance of air into the heart, to cool the same, is an important feature of the Aristotelian physiology. Beyond the Aristotelian heart, however, we cannot trace the air which enters it. Yet we find *"pneuma,"* "spirits," referred to by Aristotle, not seldom obscurely or in very general terms, as doing service, sometimes momentous service, in the physiology of generation and in certain workings within the bodies of full-grown creatures. In disease also spirits may play a very important part. These Aristotelian spirits, however, when their origin can be traced at all, are either innate or appear to be vapor produced within the body itself by heat or by disease. They do not appear to be recruited from the outer air which has penetrated the lungs and heart, that air seeming to complete its function within the lungs or within the heart itself by sustaining the native heat which is the great instrument of the soul, and in which the very soul itself is fired.[48]

Physicians of Aristotle's time, however, revived and handed on the doctrine that not only blood but a derivative of the air is distributed to the body at large through the vessels. After the distinction between veins and arteries had been clearly made and the latter had received their present name, a striking modification of this doctrine of the spirits was adopted and pressed by the Greek physician Erasistratus, about 300 B.C., not many years after the death of Aristotle. This modified doctrine separated the paths taken within the vessels by the blood and the spirits derived from the air, and declared the transmission of the necessary blood to the body at large to be by the veins only, that of the necessary spirits, styled "vital," to be by the arteries only. More than four hundred and fifty years later Galen shattered this doctrine and incorporated the vital spirits in the arteries with the blood, which he proved by epoch-making experiments to be normally present in the arteries, he, however, clearly recognizing differences between the cruder blood in the veins and the spirituous blood in the arteries. The tissues, therefore, still received vital spirits by way of the arteries, according to Galen, but not spirits in their pure gaseous Erasistratean state.[49] Now let Galen tell us more in his own words : —

"The breath from the windpipes, which had been drawn in from without, is worked up in the flesh of the lungs in the first place ; in the second place in the heart and arteries, and especially in those of the net-like plexus ; and to perfection in the ventricles of the brain, where the spirits become completely animal. But what the use may be of these animal sprits and why we have the temerity to call them so, when we confess that we are still utterly ignorant as to the substance of the anima [i.e., of the soul], this is not the moment to say." [50]

The complex physiology of this passage is so obsolete that its very phraseology is meaningless without a commentary. In the first place, what are the animal spirits? This expression, once a technical term of physiology, survives only in colloquial English, and even there merely as a label of which the origin is known to few. In this phrase the adjective "animal" does not refer to lower creatures as opposed to man, but is used in its obsolete original sense of "pertaining to the soul," for which latter the Latin word is "*anima*," the Greek word "*psyche*" (ψυχή). "Psychical spirits" would best translate into the English of to-day either the original Greek expression "*pneuma psychikon*" (πνεῦμα ψυχικόν) or its Latin equivalent "*spiritus animalis*." But the expression "animal spirits" was for too long a time an English technical term to be superseded now. These animal spirits, that is, spirits of the soul, were not peculiar to man, but were possessed by lower creatures also; for neither the Latin word "*anima*" nor the Greek word "*psyche*" implied immortality, as the English word "soul" is now so commonly understood to do. Plato formally recognized a mortal and an immortal part of the human psyche; [51] and Aristotle admitted the existence in animals lower than man of the lower grades of psyche, and conceded the lowest grade even to plants. [52] The perfected animal spirits were of the very highest physiological importance, as their name implies, they being for Galen no less than "the first instrument of the soul," [53] and thus assuming the lofty rank given by Aristotle to the native heat. For Galen the animal spirits were the medium of sensation and volition and were imparted by the ventricles of the brain to the spinal cord and nerves, the fibers of which were believed, accordingly, to consist of tubes in which the subtile animal spirits were contained, the bore of these tubes being too small to be visible.

We can now follow the quoted Galenic passage and trace the full significance of that entrance of the substance of the air into the heart which Galen repeatedly acknowledged, though sometimes grudgingly. According to Galen whatever air was taken into the heart had first been "concocted" in "the flesh of the lungs." Next, this aërial substance had been worked up in the heart with the vapor of the blood into vital spirits, and these became incorporated with the finer blood destined for the arteries. Moreover, as each arterial diastole was due to an active expansion of the arterial wall, at each diastole there became blended with the contents of the arteries still more of the substance of the air, which was sucked into the arterial skin through the countless pores of the bodily skin, these being too fine to permit bleeding. The vital spirits, thus formed and modified, were blended with the blood of the arteries and supplied to the body at large. A part of these vital spirits mounted with the blood into the carotid arteries. In the swine and the ruminants, notably in the calf, the branch given to the brain by each carotid artery breaks up at the base of the skull within the cranial cavity into numerous fine twigs, which form collectively a net-work, styled in the passage from Galen already quoted the "net-like plexus." This plexus is called by modern anatomists the *rete mirabile*. It was falsely assumed by Galen to exist in man. The plexuses of the two sides anastomose freely across the median line, and through them passes the entire blood supply of the brain; in the animals which possess them these plexuses seem the terminal branches of the vertebral arteries also. The small vessels of each net-like plexus reunite, and thus reconstitute the artery of the brain before this artery has pierced the dura mater. Galen regarded the net-like plexus as an organ of much importance intercalated in the course of the artery for the still further elaboration of the vital spirits, which, thus altered, were exhaled from the cerebral arteries into the cerebral ventricles.[54]   In these ventricles the spirits attained their final perfection, becoming "completely animal," by the aid of still more of the substance of the air, which the diastole of the pulsating brain had drawn into its cavities directly from the nares through the numerous holes in the ethmoid bones.   It is a striking fact in this connection that in some of the domestic animals on each side of the head the cavity of the nares is separated from the ventricular cavity of the brain by an exceedingly thin, though complex, partition : as may be seen on dissection, if the nares and the brain *in situ* be opened at the same time.

Now let Galen speak again as follows : —

"I have clearly shown that the brain is, in a way, the source of the animal spirits, watered and fed by inspiration and by the abundance supplied from the net-like plexus.   The proof was not so clear as to the vital spirits, but we may deem it not at all unlikely that they exist, contained in the heart and arteries, they, too, fed by respiration mainly, but to some degree by the blood also.   If there be such a thing as the natural spirits, these would be found contained in the liver and veins." [55]

The animal spirits were sustained, as we have seen, by three kinds of respiration which might be called pulmonary, cutaneous and cerebral.   We may perhaps conjecture that it was largely Galen's acceptance of the two latter, the last especially, which enabled him sometimes to treat as doubtful the entrance into the heart of that air from which the vital spirits were held to be derived.   Of the natural spirits he evidently made small account.[56]

A modern physiologist, musing upon all this, might

see in the vital spirits a dim foreshadowing of oxyhæmo-globin; might see in the operation of the animal spirits a plainer foreshadowing of the nerve impulse of to-day.

Some account, such as the foregoing, of the very complex ancient doctrine of the spirits is indispensable for the study of Harvey; for that doctrine, more or less modified, was still the accepted medical doctrine of his time. After this renewed study of the ancients let us now return again to Harvey's note-book at the place where he takes up the question of the action of the lungs upon the blood otherwise than by the cooling and ventilation of the innate heat. It is necessary in his opinion that a further concoction of the blood into spirituous arterial blood should be accomplished by the fleshy parenchyma of the lungs in animals which require a warmer, thinner, "sprightly kind of aliment," as his own English styles it.[57] The probability of such a concoction is shown by the separation of excreta which indicate it, such as sputa, at the lung.[58] On the other hand, in such creatures as frogs and turtles the lungs are fleshless, spongy, and vesicular, and give no sign of blood or excreta. Hence we may infer that the pul-monary concoction of the blood, though it probably occurs, is limited to such animals as possess fleshy and sanguinolent lungs. Hence, again, it follows that the concoction aforesaid is a function of secondary im-portance, because it is not universal; and that the foremost function of the lungs is their motion, the windpipes constituting their most important part, rather than the parenchyma.[59] Two functions of the lungs, says Harvey, are affirmed by the medical authori-ties: first, the cooling and tempering of the blood;

second, the preparation of natural spirits and air to be made into vital spirits in the heart.   From all this there result the excreta of pulmonary concoction, which are something between water and air, and the fumes which are breathed out in expiration continually and incessantly. Harvey observes correctly that Realdus Columbus had declared himself to have discovered the continual motion of the lung to be the means whereby the spirits are prepared; the blood being thinned by the agitation, thoroughly mixed with air, beaten, and prepared.[60] Harvey also cites Galen as saying that the parenchyma of the lung concocts spirits out of air as the flesh of the liver concocts the blood.[61] On turning to the Galenic passage cited by Harvey one finds that it is out of the food that the blood is thus concocted by the liver.

Realdus Columbus, to whom Harvey refers, was the Italian anatomist who in 1559, fifty-seven years before the Harveian circulation was verbally announced, gave to the world the important truth that such blood as the right ventricle imparts to the left reaches the latter by traversing the pores of the texture of the lungs,[62] instead of the pores of the septum of the ventricles, as Galen had taught. The existence of these pores of the septum Vesalius had pointedly wondered at in 1543 and had emphatically doubted in 1555.[63] Four years later his former assistant and temporary successor, Columbus, flatly denied the existence of the pores. It was natural, therefore, that in the same book in which Columbus brought forward the path through the lungs to replace that through the septum he should declare that the vital spirits are made out of air worked

up with the blood in the lungs and then merely perfected in the left ventricle. This doctrine was an
important advance beyond what Galen had taught, viz.:
that the spirits are but slightly prepared in the lungs
out of air and then sent to the left ventricle to undergo
their main preparation and to be worked up therein
with the blood which had filtered into it directly out
of the right ventricle.

So much for the views of the medical authorities.
We have found Harvey agreeing with them that the
ancient doctrine of the cooling and ventilation of the
native heat by respiration is sound. We have found
him acknowledging that in some animals some sort of
concoction also of the blood destined for the arteries
may be brought about by the pulmonary parenchyma
as a function of secondary importance. But now we
shall find him rejecting the second accepted doctrine
of the physicians, viz.: that some of the substance of
the air is taken into the pulmonary vessels and enters
the blood. This conjecture had had believers for two
thousand years, and was destined to be proved true
triumphantly after Harvey's death. In rejecting it
he threw away a precious clue to the meaning of his
own great discovery.

"It is more philosophical," he says, "not to share the common
belief that the spirits are distinct and separate from the humors
and parts because the spirits are produced in diverse places or
contained in diverse things," but to hold that the spirits and the
blood are one thing, like the cream and watery part (serum) in
milk or, to borrow a simile from Aristotle's reasonings about the
blood,[64] like heat and water in hot water, or like flame and a vapor
which feeds it (nidor). As light is to a candle, so are the spirits to
the blood. [65]

In this passage the discoverer's thought rises high, but in the next it stoops again. The next passage is headed "Spirits not from air"; and Harvey says in effect, as I understand his difficult words : —

If spirits are made by concoction out of air, the air is made either thinner or thicker in the process. If made thick, how does it get from the windpipes into the venous artery? If the spirits be thinner than air, how are they held [66] by the tunic of the lung, since this lets pass the pus and serum of empyema? [65]

In the treatise of 1628 Harvey says that Laurentius

"asserts and proves that, in empyema, serosities and pus absorbed from the cavity of the chest into the venous artery may be expelled and got rid of with the urine and fæces through the left ventricle of the heart and the arteries." [67]

Harvey's argument in his note-book continues thus : —

"How, since mixture consists in the union of altered matters, can air be thoroughly mixed and made one with blood? What is that which mixes and alters? If it be heat, the air is made thinner thereby. If it be urged that the air is thickened by cold during preparation (which is impossible in the lungs), then Aristotle's [68] argument holds good : if spirits be from the air, how about fishes, which are agile and abound in spirits?" [69]

At this point we may call to mind passages in the introduction to Harvey's treatise of 1628, published more than eleven years after he had written the notes which we are now studying. In one of these passages he speaks of what is now called the pulmonary vein, saying : —

"If it be contended that fumes and air pass to and fro by this road, as through the bronchia of the lungs, why can we find neither air nor fumes on dissection, when the venous artery has been cut out or

cut into? And how comes it that we always see the aforesaid venous artery to be full of thick blood and never of air, while we perceive that there is air remaining in the lungs?" [70]

Immediately after the foregoing passage Harvey says
that should an experimenter

"make a cut in the trachea of a living dog, forcibly fill the lungs
with air by means of a bellows and, when they have been distended,
apply a firm ligature, on opening the chest shortly after, he would
find great abundance of air in the lungs, up to their outermost
tunic, but none at all in the venous artery or in the left ventricle
of the heart. If in the living dog the heart drew air out of the
lungs or the lungs transmitted it, much more ought they to do so
in this experiment. Who, indeed, could doubt that even in a dissection, if the lungs of a dead body had been inflated, air would
enter at once, as aforesaid, did any passages exist?" [71]

Yet we have found Aristotle, more than nineteen
centuries before Harvey, recognizing that no passages
are needed for the transfer of air out of the windpipe,
and saying, of the channels from the heart, that "it is
by contact that they receive the breath [72] and transmit
it to the heart." [73]   Moreover, sixty-nine years before
Harvey's publication Columbus had repeatedly recommended the experiment of opening the venous
artery [20] in a living dog and noting that the "said
venous artery" is full of blood, not of air or fumes.
But Columbus held this observation rather to confirm
than to disprove his doctrine that the blood in the
venous artery is imbued with vital spirits derived in
the lungs from the substance of the air. Indeed, he goes
so far as to call the contents of this vessel "modified
blood and air." [74]   In this matter the earlier observer,
Columbus, shows keener insight than the later, Harvey.

Decidedly, however, the stage waits for the chemists, despite Harvey's poor opinion of them. Despite that poor opinion, too, Harvey himself turns to making chemical conjectures in the next passage of his note-book, to the study of which latter we will now return. The passage is as follows : —

"Conclusion. Opinion of W. H.

"In animals in which lungs are fleshy and full of blood these concoct the blood, seeing that spirits and blood are one thing, in the same way that the liver does and by reason of the same arguments; indeed, the lungs may rather detain fatty and oleaginous vapor by a cooling process, as oil or balsam or nutritious fat is cooled in alembic and serpentina " [75] —

"alembic" and "serpentina" answering to the "still" and "worm" of the modern distiller. Harvey, therefore, utilizes the Galenic analogy between concoction in the lungs and that of the blood and the vapors thereof, rejecting not only Galen's preliminary concoction of air into spirits in the lungs, but also Columbus's union in the lungs of blood with spirits produced in the lungs themselves out of air. Of the entrance of "the substance of air" into the blood Harvey makes emphatic denial and, by so doing, reduces the spirits either to emanations from ingredients of the body itself (thus reminding us of Aristotle), or to a mere name with which to label qualities of the blood, in treating of which he often uses the word "spirits" as a current term. Naturally, therefore, where in his lecture notes he treats of the spirits in relation to the brain and nerves his conclusions are not clearly defined, but seem consistent with his views as to the spirits in the blood, though his jotted words are not very easy to understand. On this subject he refers by name to Galen, three alternatives discussed by whom appear to be reviewed by Harvey, viz.: that sensation and motion result either from a progression from elsewhere of spirits in substance along and within the nerves; or from a vibration of spirits in substance which have their native seat within the nerves; or, lastly, from no movement of a substance, but from a transfer of "faculty" along the nerves by means of progressive qualitative alteration thereof, "such as is produced in air by the brightness of the sun." [76]   Of these three alternatives, the last seems to commend itself most to Harvey, as we should expect; the second, next; and the first, not at all; — that is, if one may so interpret the following brief passage of his lecture notes: —

"I believe that in the nerves there is no progression of spirits, but irradiation; and that the actions from which sensation and motion result are brought about as light is in air, perhaps as the flux and reflux of the sea." [77]

Also we find Harvey long years afterward saying to Riolanus: —

"Moreover, the spirits, animal, natural, vital, which dwell, contained within blind windings, in solid parts, to wit, in ligaments and nerves (especially if there be so many kinds), — these spirits are not to be regarded as so many diverse aëreal forms, nor as so many kinds of vapors." [78]

In Harvey's lecture notes the subject of respiration is brought to an end with an abrupt interrogation, which seems to reveal a sudden return of doubt as to whether too much may not have been conceded in admitting a pulmonary concoction of any sort. We read: —

"N.B. If the blood receive concoction in the lungs, why does it not traverse the lungs in the embryo?" [79]

It would seem to be Harvey's tendency to adhere to the view which limited the use of respiration entirely to the cooling and ventilation of the innate heat, by which according to ancient doctrine the heart was the central hearth, embedded in the cooling and ventilating lungs; although this ancient doctrine tallied well in most eyes with the belief that only a portion of the blood ever entered the heart at all.[80] In the first of the two Exercises which Harvey, when seventy years old, in 1649, addressed to Riolanus in defense of the circulation, the ancient respiratory cooling and ventilation take their place again as follows: —

"Thus by the aid of two extremes, viz.: cold and heat, is the temperature of the animal body retained at its mean. For as the air inspired tempers the too great heat of the blood in the lungs and centre of the body and effects the expulsion of suffocating fumes, so in its turn does the hot blood, thrown through the arteries into the entire body, cherish and nourish and keep alive all the extremities, preventing extinction due to the power of external cold." [81]

In none of the writings of his old age does Harvey deal expressly with concoction in the lungs, or more than cursorily with the entrance of the substance of air into the blood. But he repeatedly and emphatically re-affirms that blood and spirits are one thing; [82] he even declares the blood in comparison with the other parts of the body to be "possessed of powers of action beyond all the rest, and therefore, in virtue of its preëminence, meriting the title of spirit." [83] He castigates those who give the rein to overmuch speculation about the spirits. We learn that some suppose that the spirits "are engendered and are fed and increased from the thinner part of the blood"; that others suppose "the primigenial moisture" to engender and support them.[84] Then there are "those who tell us that the spirits are formed in the heart, being compounded of the vapours or exhalations of the blood (excited either by the heat of the heart or the agitation) and the inspired air"[85] — the Galenic doctrine.

"Such spirits," says Harvey of these last mentioned, "are rather to be regarded as fumes and excrementitious effluvia of the blood and body, like odours, than as natural artificers; . . . whence it seems probable also that pulmonary expiration is for the ventilation and purifying of the blood by the breathing out of these; while inspiration is in order that the blood, in passing through between the two ventricles of the heart, may be tempered by the ambient cold; lest the blood, being hot and swollen, blown up in a sort of ferment, like milk and honey boiling up, should so distend the lungs that the animal would be suffocated."[86]

As we read these words, published in Harvey's old age, we recollect the following words, written in his note-book more than thirty-three years before, viz.: "So there is cooling and ventilation of the native heat, ventilation especially."[87] We may recall also that the preservation of the native heat had sufficed to explain respiration to Harvey's ancient teacher, Aristotle, while the tenor of Aristotle's genuine works well accords with the following dictum which we have found in Harvey's note-book: "Spirits not from air." Yet the more firmly this dictum was upheld, and the more simply Aristotelian in principle did Harvey's doctrine of respiration remain, so much the less called for must have seemed that swift and endlessly repeated passage through the lungs of the whole mass of the blood, which was involved in the Harveian circulation.

In the actual phenomena of respiration, however, positive obstacles confronted the doctrine of the circulation which were harder to surmount than cobwebs of speculation, or than the mere question "*cui bono,*" which latter the steadfast observer could simply wave aside. Spirits or no spirits, there were opponents of the circulation, even in Harvey's old age, who insisted that the blood in the arteries was so different from the blood in the veins that the same blood could not be changing perpetually from arterial to venous, and *vice versa.* There was always that stubborn difference of color, plainly to be seen in man and beast, but so hard to account for in Harvey's day. Therefore, we find Harvey leaving the realm of subtleties and taking up his old weapon of demonstration, in order to minimize the differences between arterial and venous blood. Twenty years after the publication of his discovery he says to Riolanus : —

"You may also perform another experiment at the same time. If you fill two cups of the same measurement with blood, one with that which issues by leaps from an artery, the other with venous blood from a vein of the same animal, you can observe the sensible differences between the two, both immediately and later, when the blood in either cup has become coagulated and cold. This experiment will contradict those who pretend that the blood in the arteries is of one kind, that in the veins of another, on the ground that that in the arteries is more florid and seethes and is blown up with copious spirits, I know not how, like milk or honey boiling upon the fire, swelling and filling a larger space. For, were the blood which is thrown from the left ventricle of the heart into the arteries fermented thus into a frothy and flatulent condition, so that a drop or two distended the whole cavity of the aorta, unquestionably, upon the subsidence of this fermentation, the volume of the blood would return to that of a few drops,(and this is, indeed, the reason that some assign for the empty state of the arteries in the dead body); and this would be apparent in the cup which is full of arterial blood, for so we find it to happen in milk and honey when they come to cool. But if in both cups you find blood nearly of the same colour, not of very different consistency in the coagulated state, forcing out serum in the same manner and filling each cup to the same height when cold that it did when hot, this will be enough for any one to rest his faith upon, and afford argument enough, I think, for rejecting the dreams of certain people. On investigation sense and reason alike assure us that the blood of the left ventricle is not of a different kind from that of the right. . . . The blood, then, when imbued with spirits to the utmost, is not swollen with them, or fermented or blown up so as to crave and require more ample room (as can be determined with the greatest certainty on trial by the measurement of the cups); we should rather understand this blood to be possessed, after the manner of wine, of greater strength, and of an impetus to action and effectiveness, in accordance with the view of Hippocrates.

"So the blood in the arteries is the same as that in the veins; even though the former be acknowledged more spirituous and possessed of greater vital force; but the blood in the arteries is not converted into something more aëreal or rendered more vaporous; as though there were no spirits not aëreal, nor anything which gives an impetus except wind and flatulence." [88]

It is well, one may be inclined to mutter, as one reads this, but how about the color? It may be nearly the same, but certainly there is a difference. In his book "On Generation" Harvey himself describes in more detail the changes which occur in shed blood on standing, and says: "Of the red parts the upper are more florid, those below are blackish." In the same description he refers shortly after to "the florid and ruddy part which is commonly thought to be arterial blood." [89] The words last quoted evidently refer to the upper part of coagulating blood as commonly seen.   This in medical practice would be blood drawn from a vein, and Harvey says nothing of arteriotomy in this passage. Indeed, he refers in the context to venesection; and earlier in the same chapter he wrote: "Physicians observe only human blood, and this shed by venesection into a basin, and coagulated." [90]

The foregoing passages show at once that opinions had been clarified very little by the suggestive change of color caused in shed blood by contact with air. Years before, in jotting down his lecture notes, Harvey had noted that the arterial blood is redder; [91] Galen had known it; [92] it must always have been known.   In 1649 Harvey wrote: —

"Three things are especially apt to give rise to this opinion of the diversity of the blood: the first is that the blood which is drawn in arteriotomy is more florid. [93] . . . Whenever and wherever blood issues through a narrow orifice it is strained, as it were, and the thinner and lighter part, which usually swims on top and is the more penetrating, is emitted." [94]

A number of observations follow, of appearances noted in nosebleed, in the use of leeches, in cupping, and in blood-letting from veins and arteries.   All these appearances are adduced in support of the view that it is the straining of the blood which renders it more florid, and they all show that the brightening of the color of shed blood on exposure to air served only to lead Harvey off on a false scent.   Continuing he refers, as follows, to direct inspection of the dissected lungs: —

"The blood is found to be much more florid within the lungs and after it is squeezed out of them, than in the arteries." [95]

A few pages farther on he states, categorically, the false conclusion to which he has been driven, saying : —

"It is no less plain why the blood of the lungs is so ruddy; for it is thinner, because there it is filtered through." [96]

Nothing indicates better Harvey's readiness to minimize the essential differences between venous and arterial blood than a passage in the treatise of 1628, in which he says that, compared with the left ventricle, the right ventricle "is of greater capacity, that it may supply not only matter to the left ventricle, but also nourishment to the lungs." [97]   It should be remembered that, in Harvey's day, the so-called bronchial arteries were still unknown, through which the tissues of the lungs are supplied with arterial blood from the aorta.[98] Not only Columbus,[99] but even Galen,[100] had each devised an erroneous way in which to provide the lungs with "spirituous" or "vital" blood, in addition to the venous blood from the right ventricle; but Harvey is obviously content to let the latter suffice for their nutrition.

What has gone before indicates how erroneous it is to speak of the pulmonary transit, as Columbus had set it forth in 1559, nineteen years before Harvey's birth, as though Columbus were in some sort a sharer in the discovery of the circulation. Those who so speak fail to note the difference between blood and *the* blood. Although Columbus girded at Galen and corrected him, Columbus's pulmonary transit of a fraction of the blood by curing more than one defect of the

Galenic doctrine strengthened the erroneous Galenic physiology of the blood-movement. Of these larger features Columbus not only was no enemy, but remained a devoted adherent. His doctrine certainly paved the way for Harvey's, but in no more immediate sense than did Galen's doctrine that blood is naturally contained in the arteries.[80]

Indeed, Harvey categorically stated that the movement of blood through the lungs had nothing to do with his discovery. In a Latin letter from London written in 1651 to P. M. Slegel in Hamburg, Harvey says in his old age : —

"Meantime, as Riolanus uses his utmost efforts to oppose the passage of blood into the left ventricle through the lungs, and brings it all hither through the septum, and so vaunts himself as having upset the very foundation of the Harveian circulation, (although I have nowhere laid that down as a foundation for my circulation ; for the blood fetches a circuit in very many red-blooded animals in which no lungs are to be found), it may be well here to relate an experiment which I lately tried in the presence of several of my colleagues, and from the cogency of which there is no escape."[101]

The parenthesis certainly is a striking one.

No less striking is the last word published by Harvey about respiration. We have heard him deny the entrance of air into the blood and doubt the occurrence of any concoction in the lungs. Now we shall hear him throw over even the cooling of the innate heat, a respiratory doctrine to which he has seemed hitherto to hold with conviction. In the essay "On Parturition" published in 1651 with the treatise "On Generation," he says : —

"In the meantime I would propose this question to the learned : How comes it that the fœtus continues in its mother's womb after the seventh month? If brought forth at that time it breathes at will, indeed could not survive one little hour without breathing; yet, as I have said, if it remain in the womb it keeps alive and well beyond the ninth month without the aid of respiration. . . . Whoso shall attend carefully to these things and consider more closely the nature of air, will, I think, readily grant that air is given to animals neither for cooling nor as nutriment; for it is a fact that after the fœtus has once drawn breath it may be suffocated more quickly than when entirely excluded from the air; as though heat were unkindled by air within the fœtus rather than allayed. Thus much, merely by the way, on the subject of respiration; perhaps I shall treat of it more fully in its proper place. Surely a more knotty subject could hardly be found, as the arguments on both sides are very evenly balanced." [102]

So we find Harvey in his old age induced by lifelong study to question, if not deny, even the cooling effects of respiration, and to end with a practical confession of ignorance. Instead, therefore, of the circulation and its swiftness being explained by the urgent need of "the substance of the air" experienced by certain tissues, that movement of the whole mass of the blood through the lungs, which was so novel a physiological fact, does not seem to have affected his view of the problems of respiration. Nor could he properly explain the respiratory change in the color of the blood, which seemed to support the ancient doctrine that the blood is of two different kinds. Since he could not invoke respiration to elucidate the circulation and its rapidity, and since he himself declared that such rapidity could not be needed for the simple feeding of the tissues, what was left to be invoked? It is no wonder that eight years [103] after the publication of his discovery Harvey denied that he had ever seriously undertaken to explain the use of the circulation; that at the end of thirteen years more he repeated this denial in his old age; [104] although he had not refrained from expressing such conjectures as must always be evoked in the mind of a great observer by a discovery of the first importance made by himself. Yet the phenomena of the very circulation used were so striking as to cry aloud for elucidation; for Harvey's own clinching statement that the heart drives into the aorta at least one thousand drachms of blood in half an hour,[105] this *reductio ad absurdum*, which cut the ground from under the feet of his opponents, left him helpless in his turn to account for the need of so huge a flooding of the arteries.

Since it was not to be swiftly altered in the lungs that the whole mass of the blood hurried back from all parts of the chest, what then?

CHAPTER IV

THE CIRCULATION AND THE ARISTOTELIAN PRIMACY OF THE HEART

IT has been stated already that the first announcement of the circulation is to be found in Harvey's lecture notes. The following is the text of the memorable passage in question, which I have translated from Harvey's Latin. He says: —

"It is proved by the structure of the heart that the blood is perpetually transferred through the lungs into the aorta, as by two clacks of a water-bellows to rayse water. It is proved by the ligature that there is a transit of the blood from the arteries to the veins; whereby it is demonstrated that a perpetual movement of the blood in a circle is brought about by the beat of the heart. Is this for the sake of nutrition, or of the better preservation of the blood and members by infusion of heat, the blood in turn being cooled by heating the members and heated by the heart?" [106]

The words "as by two clacks of a water-bellows to rayse water" are Harvey's own racy English, embedded in his Latin text. The "ligature" is the flat band which is tied about the upper arm when bleeding from a vein is to be practised at the bend of the elbow. The Hippocratic physicians called this band a *"taenia,"* [107] and even in their day it was known to hasten the flow of blood from the opened vein when applied as above stated, but yet to check the flow if tied too tight. This

42

Page 80, right, of William Harvey's *Prelectiones Anatomiæ Universalis*, or Lecture Notes of 1616. The passage contains the first recorded mention of the movement of the blood in a circle.

WH conſtat per fabricam cordis ſanguinem
per pulmones in Aortam perpetuo
tranſferri, as by two clacks of a
water bellows to rayſe water
conſtat per ligaturam tranſitum ſanguinis
ab arterijs ad venas
vnde Δ perpetuum ſanguinis motum
in circulo fieri pulſu cordis
An ? hoc gratia Nutritionis
an magis Conſervationis ſanguinis
et Membrorum per Infuſionem calidam
viciſſimque ſanguis Calefaciens
membra frigifactum a Corde
Calefit

Transcript of the preceding page.

clinical observation had awaited a rational explanation
for more than nineteen centuries.[108]

Our most immediate interest in the foregoing passage
lies in this: that on the very same page, with the few
clear simple words which tell for the first time of Harvey's facts and proofs, he has briefly written down conjectures as to the meaning of the circulation.   These are
as strikingly put as certain jottings are obscure which
deal on a neighboring page with some possible meanings
of the heart-beat.[109]   In neither group of conjectures
do the functions of the lungs play a part; but the discoverer asks himself whether it be not to revisit the
heat of the heart that the whole mass of the blood
circles back to the chest in its Harveian course!   More
than thirty-two years after the date of Harvey's note-
book Harvey wrote to Riolanus: —

"There are some who consider that as no impulsion of nutriment is required for the nutrition of plants, their particles attract-
ing little by little whatever they need to replace what they have
lost, so in animals there is no need of any impulsion, the vegetative faculty in both working alike. But there is a difference. In
animals a perpetual flow of warmth is required to cherish the members, to keep them alive by the aid of vivifying heat, and to restore
parts injured from without. It is not merely nutrition that needs
to be provided for." [110]

In the first Exercise to Riolanus Harvey had touched
also upon the use of the circulation, interweaving this
doctrine of heat with the doctrine of respiration as he
then held it, in a passage the last part of which I have
quoted already.   Quoted more fully he says: —

"And this, indeed, is the principal use and end of the circulation, for which the blood revolves with perpetual influence in its

ceaseless course and is driven along its circuit: namely, that all the parts in dependence upon the blood may be kept alive by the primary innate heat and in their state of vital and vegetative being, and may perform all their functions; whilst, to use the language of physiologists, they are sustained and actuated by the inflowing heat and vital spirits. Thus by the aid of two extremes, viz.: cold and heat, is the temperature of the animal body retained at its mean. For as the air inspired tempers the too great heat of the blood in the lungs and center of the body and effects the expulsion of suffocating fumes, so in its turn does the hot blood, thrown through the arteries into the entire body, cherish and nourish and keep alive all the extremities, preventing extinction due to the power of external cold." [111]

"The innate fire is not in the right ventricle," a Hippocratic author had written, who had written also that the wall of the left ventricle is dense, to guard the strength of the heat.[112]   Aristotle, too, had placed in the heart the "origin" of the "natural innate heat"; [113] had likened the heart to "the hearth on which shall lie the natural kindling, well protected also, as being the acropolis of the body." [114]   At a later day Galen had affirmed the same doctrine.[115]

Let us turn now to the famous treatise of 1628, published twelve years after the note-book had been written. In the chapter in which Harvey says "I tremble lest I have mankind at large for my enemies" and then publishes and names the circulation, — in this chapter, before passing to his proofs, he published the following words which resound in a way very different from the simplicity of the note-book : —

"So probably it may come to pass in the body through the movement of the blood that all the parts are nourished, cherished, quickened, by the hotter, perfected, vaporous, spirituous, and, so to speak, alimentive blood; that the blood, on the other hand, is cooled, coagulated, and rendered, as it were, effete in the parts; whence it returns to its origin, namely, the heart, as to its fountain, or the hearth of the body, to regain perfection. There by the potent and fervid natural heat, a treasury of life, as it were, the blood is liquefied anew and becomes pregnant with spirits and, so to speak, with balsam. Thence the blood is distributed again; and all this depends upon the motion and pulsation of the heart.

"The heart, therefore, is the origin of life and the sun of the microcosm, even as the sun in his turn might well be called the heart of the world; by the vigor and pulsation of the heart the blood is moved, perfected, quickened, and delivered from corruption and thickening; and the function of nourishing, cherishing, quickening the entire body is performed by that intimate hearth, the heart, the foundation of life, the author of all. But of these matters more conveniently when I shall speculate as to the final cause of motion such as this." [116]

Upon this florid passage follow the classic six chapters which bring forward with such power and calm the proofs of the circulation. These are succeeded in their turn by words which echo their sobriety, as follows: —

"It will not be beside the question to show also from certain familiar reasonings, that the circulation is both convenient and necessary. In the first place, since death is corruption from deficiency of heat [117] and since all living things are warm, all dying things cold, the heat requires a seat and origin, a home and hearth, as it were, in which the tinder of nature, the first beginning of the innate fire, may be contained and preserved; a place from which, as from their origin, heat and life may flow out into all the parts, whence nutriment may come and upon which concoction and nutrition and all quickening may depend. That this place is the heart, that this is the origin of life as aforesaid, I should hope that none would doubt.

"Hence the blood has need of motion, of motion such that it may return to the heart; for, if sent to the outer parts of the body, far from its source,[118] and left unmoved, it would become coagulated. Heat and spirits are seen to be generated and preserved in all by motion, to vanish if quiet supervene. Therefore, the blood, thickened or stiffened by the cold of the extremities and of the ambient [air] and destitute of spirits, as in the dead, must needs return to its source and origin in order to keep itself whole, to seek thence and repair again its heat and spirits." [119] . . .

"Moreover," Harvey says, a page farther on, "since all animals live by nutriment concocted in their interior, it is necessary that the concoction and distribution thereof be perfect; and, further, that a place and receptacle exist where the nutriment may be perfected and whence it may be led off to the several members. Now this place is the heart, for it alone of all the parts contains blood for the public use in its cavities, the auricles and ventricles, as in cisterns and storehouse; not merely blood for its private use in the coronary vein and artery." [120]

In the next chapter we obtain glimpses of the pathological relations of this physiology. Harvey brings forward tertian fever as a case in point, explaining that the febrile paroxysm is produced when

"the preternatural heat which has been kindled in the heart is diffused throughout the entire body by way of the arteries, together with the morbific matter which thus is evaporated and dissolved by nature." [121]

As a student of the Greek science reads the foregoing passages, he clearly sees that the new wine of the circulating blood is poured into the old bottles of the Aristotelian physiology; and Harvey tells us so himself, in the last chapter of his most famous treatise. He says : —

"No less should we agree with Aristotle as to the sovereignty of the heart, in dealing with the following and similar questions : Does it receive motion and sensation from the brain, blood from the liver; or is it the origin of the veins and of the blood? For they who try to refute him leave out, or do not grasp, the main argument, which is that the heart is the first part to exist and has in it blood, life, sensation, motion, before the brain or the liver has been made or is clearly to be distinguished, or at least before either can perform any function. So the heart with its own proper organs constructed for motion — as it were, an internal animal — is the earlier formed; and, this being the first made part, it is the will of nature that thereafter the entire animal be made, nourished, preserved, perfected by the heart to be its achievement and abode. The heart is governor everywhere, like the chief in a commonwealth with whom is lodged the first and highest authority. In an animal all power is derived from and depends upon the heart as its origin and foundation." [122]

The main argument, which is that the heart is the first part to exist, is simply the argument from the development of the embryo in the hen's egg. The study of this development day by day had been recommended by one of the Hippocratic writers,[123] and Aristotle had laid stress upon the changes in the embryo during incubation.[124] Harvey, in his turn, had studied them carefully. The ancients could have made their observations only with the naked eye, but Harvey had the aid of a simple lens, though of nothing approaching in power to a microscope.[125] In the treatise of 1628 he speaks as follows of what he thus observed : —

"If you turn to the formation of the chick in the egg, the first thing to exist therein, as I have said, is a mere vesicle, or auricle, or pulsating drop of blood. Afterward, when growth has gone on, the heart is completed. . . . In a hen's egg after four or five days of incubation I have shown the visible presence of the rudiment of the chick in the form of a little cloud; in an egg, that is, which had been immersed in clear tepid water after removal of the shell. In the middle of the aforesaid little cloud there was a palpitating bloody point, so fine that in contracting it disappeared and became invisible, but reappeared on its relaxation, looking like the point of a needle, and of a ruddy color; so that being now visible and now invisible, as though now existent and now non-existent, it evinced palpitation and the beginning of life." [126]

In the same treatise Harvey promises to publish more observations

"on the formation of the fœtus, where numerous problems of the following order can find a place: Why should this point be made or perfected earlier, that later? As regards the dominance of the members: Which part is the cause of the other? There are very many problems connected with the heart, such as: Why should it be the first thing (as Aristotle says in his third book on the parts of animals) [127] to acquire consistency, and be seen possessed of life, motion, and sensation, before anything has been perfected in the rest of the body? And in like manner regarding the blood: Why is it before all, and how possessed of the beginnings [128] of life and of the animal, and of the craving to move and be impelled hither and thither, to which end the heart would seem to have been made?" [129]

In Harvey's celebrated treatise, despite various frank questionings by the way, such as that just quoted about the blood, he so frankly follows in the footsteps of "the master of them that know" that Aristotle need not be cited at length to prove the fact. To Aristotle are largely due Harvey's references to the heart as the central source of indispensable vital heat; his references to aliment perfected in the heart; his blending of psychological doctrines with the doctrine of the movement of the blood. Therefore, a brief account of how this became possible will be germane.

When an ancient observer looked with the naked eye at the very early embryo of the fowl, he distinguished at first only a blood-red point, which pulsated, or "leapt." This Aristotle judged to be the heart, containing blood before any blood-vessel had shown itself and before blood was visible in any other part. Very soon, however, two vessels containing blood were seen, according to him, to extend from the rudimentary heart toward the periphery. From these and other considerations Aristotle inferred that both the blood and all its containing vessels owe their first origin to the heart; and that throughout life the liquid made elsewhere from the food enters the heart, there to be perfected into blood by the action of the vital innate heat, of which, as we have seen, he held the fiery central hearth to be within the heart. Naturally, therefore, he believed the blood not to be hot of itself, but to acquire its vivifying heat at the heart, the pulsation of which he held to be caused directly by the seething of the blood within. When thus perfected and charged with heat the blood, according to him, is distributed from the heart through the vena cava as well as the aorta. These great vessels and their subdivisions Aristotle distinguished anatomically; but he made no serious physiological distinction between what we call the veins and the arteries, and, himself, applied the word "artery" to the windpipe only. As to the cavities and contents of the heart, even as to the number of its cavities, he had obscure, complex, and erroneous ideas, and of the valves he knew nothing. He recognized no essential differences between the matters distributed by way of the vena cava and by way of the aorta, all being, alike, one thing, blood; though the blood was hotter or cooler, thinner or thicker, purer or cruder, in different regions or parts of the body, in different sets of vessels, in different cavities of the heart, or at different times in the same place.

We have seen already that, in the genuine works of Aristotle, there is no sign that what we call the tissues of the adult require or receive a derivative of the air, whether crudely mingled with the blood in the earlier Hippocratic way, or separate in Erasistratean fashion, or in the form of such "spirituous blood" as Galen afterward accepted. We have seen that the air which Aristotle believed to enter the heart for cooling purposes, cannot be traced beyond it; that whatever spirits may exist in the body for him, would seem to be either of the nature of vapor produced within the body itself, or of a nature quite indeterminate.[130]

The living egg of the hen has had a vast deal to do with the history of psychology as well as of physiology. It is partly owing to what Aristotle believed to go on in the egg that we speak to-day of good hearts and bad hearts — even of sweethearts. Aristotle knew nothing of the nerves, and, therefore, could reasonably fail to find conclusive evidence that the brain and spinal cord had to do with what we call nervous functions. So he fell back upon a doctrine at least as old as the Iliad,[131] and made a psychological center of the heart. This being proved, for Aristotle, largely by its demeanor in the early embryo, to be the life-long source of the nutritive blood; and being, for him, the central hearth of the heat by means of which the blood is perfected and warmed; he held it a matter of necessity that in the heart should dwell the so-called "nutritive soul"; that is, the faculty which uses as its most immediate instrument the "innate," "natural," "vital," "psychical," heat, to bring about nutrition, growth, and generation. He says: —

"It is impossible that the other faculties of the soul should exist without the nutritive, or these without the natural fire; for in this has nature set that faculty aglow." [132]

Dealing with these other faculties, he sees that there must be an organ where the results of sight, hearing, and the other senses, are compared; and deliberately discussing and rejecting the claims made for the brain he makes the heart this "common sense-organ of all the sense-organs," as he styles it.   He says: —

"If in all the creatures the seat of life is in this part, it is clear that here also must the origin of sensation be; for we say that the body has life because it is an animal, but we say that it is animal because it has sensation." [133]

Less hollow rings the argument in the modern ear, when the ancient thinker bases it on conclusions drawn from observation.   We learn from him that only those parts are sensitive which contain blood, as opposed to hair and nails, or even to the blood, if taken by itself. We learn, therefore, that as the heart of the embryo is the first part to contain blood, it is the first part to be sensitive and hence is the central source of sensation. Moreover, Aristotle, like Plato,[134] knowing nothing of the nerves, judges the blood-vessels to be sensory paths; and blood-vessels connect, not only the sensitive flesh, but all the more special sense-organs with the heart.   Such is the outline of the reasons why Aristotle held the heart to be the lifelong seat, not only of the "nutritive soul," but of the "sensory soul" as well.

Pain, pleasure, and desire would naturally dwell beside sensation in the heart, which Aristotle held to be obviously the seat of the emotions, as proved by its

palpitation when they are stirred. Moreover, it is
desire, seated in the heart, which incites to action, to
motion, movement thus resulting from sensation; and,
in general, "the movements" of every sense both begin
and end at the heart; the word here translated "movement" [135] being used, in the technical diction of Aristotle,
to include not only the "molar motion" of modern parlance, but also subtle forms of change of state. Further,
in the early embryo the heart itself is plainly the first
part which possesses motion; it visibly taking the
lead in this, moving "as though itself an animal."
The pulsating movements of the heart are the direct
effects of the seething and vaporization within it;
while, in the respiratory movements, the chest wall
is pushed out by an expansion due to the vital heat,
whose cardiac hearth the lungs inclose, and then
follows inward a contraction due to the cooling air
which has been drawn into the expanding lungs. As
the bodily movements, in general, are "brought about
by drawing and slackening" and originate at the heart,
it is appropriate that the heart contains tendinous
structures [136] within itself; "for it needs the service
and strength" of such. [137] It is too, in a sense, the
origin of the discontinuous tendinous and ligamentous
structures of the body. Aristotle's doctrine of the
heart as the source of motion seems especially vague.
But, hardy thinker though he was, he scarcely could be
definite on this subject, even in speculation. He knew
that heat expands and cold contracts: he recognized
the force which, as he believed, confined or compressed
vapor exerts in living bodies, not only in health but in
disease; and he knew the strength imparted to bodily

effort by holding the breath. His genuine writings, however, bring forward no *modus operandi*, except in the case of respiration and of the movements of the heart itself. We are given no inkling as to how the tendons are normally drawn and slackened in obedience to the will, for the true function of muscle was unknown to Aristotle (Harvey to the contrary notwithstanding),[138] and the blood-vessels were the only continuous special paths between center and periphery which Aristotle could make out. In his time, as we have seen, the nerves had not been distinguished, even anatomically, from the bands and cords of the ligaments and tendons.

So, for Aristotle, the nutritive, sensory, and motor faculties, the desires and emotions, in short all the souls or parts of the soul (to use the ancient phraseology) that are not the most exalted, dwell in fire within the heart, suitably and honorably placed at the central "acropolis." To the divine mind of man, on the other hand, he does not assign a definite special dwelling-place within the body.

Harvey differed often and widely from Aristotle. Yet even in his old age he wrote: "The authority of Aristotle has always such weight with me that I never think of differing from him inconsiderately." [139] Cannot one fancy, may not one conjecture, that in the eyes of the discoverer of the circulation his great discovery, fundamental, new, and original, as he rightly claimed it to be, may at times have seemed to constitute a thorough correcting and filling in of a rough sketch dashed off at the Lyceum? Let us see.

Aristotle had no conception of anything resembling a circulation of the blood, nor any definite mechanical ideas as to its movement. While the vena cava as well as the aorta received blood from his valveless heart and yielded it to the body at large, blood ebbed back to the heart during sleep, and the warm nutrient liquid which the vena cava and the aorta yielded to the tissues had previously entered the heart continuously but in an imperfect state through both of these great vessels, to go forth again through both, perfected into blood and heated, with no perplexing differences of color noted between that in the great vein and that in the aorta. The relations between the food, the blood, the heart, and the body at large, though recognized to be complex, may well have presented themselves to Aristotle with something of the vagueness with which the relations between the food, the liquids, the contractile vacuole, and the living substance of a protozoön, present themselves to us. If the heart, retaining its Aristotelian powers, were found to receive the blood imperfect or impaired, but to receive it by the veins only, and to send it out, but only by the arteries, warmed and perfected or restored to perfection at its Aristotelian source ; what have we but the systemic part of the circulation, as it may have pictured itself sometimes to Harvey? [140]

CHAPTER V

THUS it is striking to find Harvey, as the champion
against Galen of a view essentially Aristotelian, entering
the field of controversy where ancient Greek still met
ancient Greek in the modern Europe of 1628.

The discoveries of the nerves and the valves of the
heart had made great difficulties for the Aristotelian
psychology and physiology shortly after Aristotle's
time. We have seen that the semilunar valves were
described, and their use noted, in a treatise included in
the Hippocratic collection; [141] and all the valves, both
arterial and auriculo-ventricular, were well recognized
by Erasistratus, whose acquaintance we have made
already, and who flourished about 300 B.C., Aristotle
having died in 322 B.C. Erasistratus, we remember,
was more than four centuries earlier than Galen and
more than nineteen centuries earlier than Harvey.

That the heart throughout life is not only the source
of the perfected blood, but gives out blood to the vena
cava for distribution, had been rendered a hard saying,
especially by the recognition of the tricuspid valve.[142]
Galen, however, like the somewhat earlier Greek
physician Aretæus, the Cappadocian,[143] was not confronted by this difficulty, for they both adhered to an
ancient doctrine to be found in the Hippocratic treatise

"On Nourishment," and there sketched with mingled clearness and vagueness in the following pithy saying :—

"Root of the veins, the liver; root of the arteries, the heart. Out of these wander into all parts blood and spirits, and through these heat comes in." [144]

Obviously the doctrine here foreshadowed was quite irreconcilable with the views of Aristotle.

In studying the works of Harvey and of his contemporaries and predecessors it must be borne in mind that, from ancient times past the time of Harvey to more modern days, the word "heart" was very commonly used by physicians and men of science to mean simply the ventricular mass, without the auricles, which were reckoned in with the great vessels. In slaughter-houses the word is still used in this ancient sense. Harvey's practice was fluctuating; for the word is used by him sometimes to mean the ventricular mass only, sometimes, as in the science of to-day, to mean the ventricular mass and the auricles taken together.

According to the more detailed views of Galen and his school the blood was perfected and had its central source not in the heart, but in the liver, to which the portal vein brought a cruder liquid derived from the products of digestion. In the liver the veins also originated, while the arteries originated at the heart. The blood left its source in the liver, by way of the roots of the venous system, that is, by the hepatic veins of modern anatomy. From these it entered the great venous trunk, the vena cava, a vessel which comprised the inferior cava, the right auricle, and the superior cava of our present nomenclature. Upon

leaving the liver the blood at once divided into two
sharply diverging streams, one flowing directly downward through the vena cava, the belly, and the lower
extremities; the other stream flowing directly upward
through the vena cava to the chest, the upper extremities, and the head.   Therefore, that part of the vena
cava which we call the right auricle simply formed a
part of the upward pathway of the blood, at a place
where some of the blood left this upward pathway and
flowed through a side opening into the right ventricle.
This ventricle, therefore, received only a fraction of that
portion of the blood which ascended from the liver.
The rest of the ascending blood mounted in the vena
cava past the right opening which led into the ventricle
and, having traversed thus what we call the right
auricle, entered and traversed what we call the superior
vena cava, to be distributed to the veins and tissues
of the arms and head.   Of the fraction of the blood
that entered the right ventricle a part went to the lungs
simply for their nutrition, by the "arterial vein" —
the pulmonary artery of modern parlance — and a part
percolated in a refined condition through pores of the
septum from the right ventricle to the left, to be worked
up there with the vital spirits and thus become the
basis of the spirituous blood of the arteries.   From the
left ventricle this spirituous blood went to the body
at large by way of the arteries.   There is no evidence
that Galen believed any blood to pass from the right
to the left ventricle otherwise than through the pores
of the septum.   As he says, however, that the branches
of the "venous artery" (our pulmonary vein) "transmit
thin and pure and vaporous blood in abundance" to

the lungs for their nutrition,[145] we may infer that he held this supply to be derived from the left ventricle like that of the rest of the body. This was possible, according to Galen's system, because he held to the irrational opinion that what is now called the mitral valve closed less perfectly than the other valves, inasmuch as it possessed only two segments instead of three.

This supposed imperfection of the mitral valve played an important part in Galen's system, for it was possible thereby for the lung to receive, not only some spirituous blood from the left ventricle of the heart, but also, and especially, the injurious fumes which Galen held to arise from combustion in the left ventricle, to escape into the venous artery past the imperfect mitral valve, and to be exhaled in expiration. When this valvular door was open, therefore, the left ventricle drew from the lungs into itself crude spirits, these to be returned in some part perhaps to the lungs as spirituous blood in company with the deleterious fumes, when the valvular door was only ajar. This imperfection of the valve of two segments, however, was but a constant and fortunate exaggeration of a condition shared to a slight degree by all the valves; for Galen held these, in the act of closing, to allow slight regurgitation of spirits, vapor, or even of blood; and to do so exceptionally even when closed, if the movement of the heart were of unusual force. He commonly, however, assumed the tricuspid, pulmonary, and aortic valves to be competent, especially if he could gain a polemical point by doing so.[146]

More than thirteen centuries later Columbus, as we have learned, announced that blood from the right ventricle entered the left ventricle, not by pores of the septum, but exclusively by pores of the lungs, in passing through which latter it became spirituous blood, needing but little elaboration in the ventricle before entering the arteries for distribution to the body.   Columbus denied and derided the passage of fumes from the left ventricle to the lungs, while he accepted the ancient doctrine of the cooling effect of respiration.   His view of the meaning of the pulmonary transit is therefore a striking approximation to the truth — a closer one than that of Harvey, who questioned everything except the fumes given off in expiration, which fumes, of course, Harvey did not send along the Galenic path.   As Columbus declared the spirituous blood to be made up in the lungs, and these, therefore, to need no supply thereof from the left ventricle; and as he also denied the passage of fumes through the venous artery; the flow through the latter became simplified, spirituous blood alone passing through it, and in the true direction from the lungs to the heart.   Accordingly the mitral valve also was cured of its Galenic imperfection; to the latter Columbus does not even refer, but he simply describes all the four valves as competent.

Columbus, therefore, set forth the true course, and in no small degree the true nature and meaning, of the movement whereby blood passes from the right auriculo-ventricular ring to the aorta, and in so doing he expelled important errors from the Galenic system. But, strange. to say, by thus purging it he greatly strengthened it, as was mentioned earlier in this paper, for he harmonized the fundamental doctrine of the

Galenic system with the true mechanism and working of the cardiac valves, and with a rational theory of respiration.[147] This fundamental Galenic doctrine was the direct distribution of blood to the tissues through the veins from the liver as a center; no more than a fraction of the blood ever passing the tricuspid valve to reach the lungs or to enter the arteries as spirituous blood. Of this doctrine Columbus was not only an adherent, but a warm partisan against the Aristotelians; and, like Galen more than thirteen centuries before, Columbus points with emphasis to the tricuspid valve as evidence of the falsity of the Aristotelian doctrine that crude blood enters the heart to be perfected and returned thence to the vena cava for distribution.[148] The Galenic view that the liver is the origin of the veins and the source of the blood, by which word, unqualified, was meant the venous blood, was known even down to Harvey's day as the view of "the physicians," as opposed to that of "the philosophers," who contended in ingenious ways for the view of the great philosopher Aristotle that the heart is the origin of the veins and the source of the blood.   Harvey in this contest repeatedly ranges himself in his writings with the Aristotelians and against the Galenists;[149] we shall see him bring the circulation into play to give very effective aid to the former against Galen himself.

Bearing in mind the Galenic meaning of the word "blood," and remembering that, in spite of the weak points in Galen's own armor, he possessed in the tricuspid valve a formidable weapon against the followers of Aristotle, listen to the following passage from Harvey's treatise of 1628. He says : —

"Whether or no the heart imparts anything more to the blood than transposition, locomotion, and distribution, whether it imparts heat also, or spirits, or perfection, must be looked into later and gathered from other observations. For the present be it enough to have shown sufficiently that during the beat of the heart the blood is transfused and withdrawn from the veins into the arteries through the ventricles of the heart, and is distributed to the body at large.

"This, to be sure, is conceded by all after a fashion, it being gathered from the structure of the heart and the arrangement, position, and use of the valves. But they seem to waver blindly as though in a dark place, and they put together varied, incoherent, and more or less contradictory doctrines and, indeed, set forth much upon conjecture, as has been shown already.

"There seems to me to have been one single principal cause of hesitation and error in this matter, viz.: the connection between the heart and the lung in man. The disappearance of the arterial vein in the lungs having been noted, and likewise that of the venous artery, great obscurity prevailed as to whence or how the right ventricle distributed the blood to the body, or the left ventricle drew blood from the vena cava. This is attested by the words of Galen when he inveighs against Erasistratus regarding the origin and use of the veins and the coction of the blood. 'You will answer,' Galen says, 'that the way of it is this: that the blood is prepared beforehand in the liver and is transferred thence to the heart to receive the rest of its proper character in complete perfection. Surely this does not seem devoid of reason; for no great and perfect work can be accomplished suddenly at one attempt and receive its entire polish from a single instrument. If then this be so, show us another vessel which leads the completely perfected blood forth from the heart, and distributes it to the whole body as the artery does the spirits.' [150] Behold Galen disapproving and putting aside a reasonable opinion because, besides not seeing the path of transit, [151] he cannot find a vessel to distribute the blood from the heart to the whole body!

"But had there been anyone on the spot to take the part of Erasistratus or of that opinion which is now our own and is confessed by Galen himself to be reasonable in other respects; and had the person aforesaid pointed his finger at the great artery [aorta] as the distributer of the blood from the heart to the body at large, — I wonder what answer that divine man would have made, full of genius and of learning as he was! Had he said that the artery distributed spirits and not blood, he certainly would sufficiently have refuted Erasistratus, who believed that only spirits were contained in the arteries; but in so doing Galen would have contradicted himself and would shamefully have denied what he sharply contends to be true in a special book [152] which he wrote against that same Erasistratus. For he proves by many powerful arguments, and demonstrates by experiments, that blood, and not spirits, is naturally contained in the arteries.

"But since the divine man concedes, as he often does in that same place, 'that all the arteries of the body arise from the great artery, and this from the heart; and that for a certainty blood is naturally contained and borne onward in all of them,' he maintaining 'that the three sigmoid valves placed at the orifice of the aorta forbid the return of blood into the heart, and that nature would never have set these valves in apposition to the most preëminent of the viscera were the valves not to do it some most important service;' — since, I say, the father of physicians concedes all this and in these very words, as he does in the book aforesaid, I do not see how he can deny that the great artery is the vessel adapted to distribute the blood, now arrived at complete perfection, from the heart to the body at large." [153]

Thus does the great English discoverer bring the pulmonary transit and the circulation of the blood to the rescue of the Aristotelian heart, despite Galen and the tricuspid valve! Between Harvey and the school that refused to the heart more than a fraction of the blood, there could be no peace. It is the Galenists whose system he attacked and shattered so thoroughly; and those who long and bitterly opposed the acceptance of the Harveian circulation were of the Galenic school. In a private letter written twenty-three years after the

publication of his discovery, Harvey excuses the
French physician Riolanus for having slighted the circulation not long before, saying, among other things : —

"It was proper that the dean of the College of Paris should
keep the medicine of Galen in repair ; and should admit no novel-
ties into his school without the utmost winnowing." [154]

CHAPTER VI

WE have found the discoverer of the circulation an admirer and defender of Aristotle; but we shall leave him far less Aristotelian than we found him. Before he died, he had transferred to the blood itself that physiological primacy which Aristotle had given to the heart; Harvey having come to regard the blood even as the very seat of the soul, harking back to a Greek doctrine older than Aristotle and expressly discountenanced by him.[155] This final view of Harvey was not simply an outcome of his old age, though he develops and formally declares and insists upon the doctrine of the primacy of the blood in the writings which he published when beyond the age of seventy, more than twenty years after the publication of his treatise of 1628. We have seen that in this his most famous work he adheres impressively to the Aristotelian doctrine of the primacy of the heart; though even this work contains utterances of Harvey which do not well accord with that doctrine. More than eleven years earlier, when making notes for his lectures of 1616, he asked himself in striking terms, whether the circulation do not exist in order that the blood may be heated by the heart.[156] Yet there are passages in those very same notes which show that, beside vaguer conjectures,[157] the doctrine of the primacy of the blood was present clearly to Harvey's mind even so early as in his thirty-seventh year. In his lecture notes four passages are especially significant as to this doctrine. Of these the first is as follows : —

> "Yf I could shew what I hav seene, yᵗ weare att an end between physicians et philosophers."

After these words in English Harvey falls into his usual Latin, which may be translated thus : —

> "For the blood is rather the author of the viscera than they of it, because the blood is present before the viscera, nor yet coming from the mother,[158] for in the egg there is a drop. The soul [159] is in the blood." [160]

In a second passage of his note-book Harvey says, speaking of the heart : —

> "It is most exceeding full of contained blood, as no other viscus is. Wherefore Aristotle [holds] against the physicians that the origin of the blood is not in the liver but in the heart, because in the liver there is no blood outside the veins. Rather is the blood the origin of both, as I have seen." [161]

In a third passage Harvey says of the heart that its

> "temperature is exceeding hot, inasmuch as it is exceeding full of blood." [162]

In a fourth passage of the lecture notes which bears upon the primacy of the blood we may read : —

> "1. [The heart] is the most principal part of all, not because of itself,[163] for its flesh is more fibrous and harder and colder than the liver, but because of the abundance of blood and spirits in the ventricles.
>
> "1. Whence the fount of the entire heat.

* * * * * * *

> "Whence the auricles pulsate, after removal of the heart, because of the multitudinous blood.[164]

"2. Nor is [the heart] the principal part because of its origin: for I believe that the ventricles (which in the fœtus are both united as in fishes) are made out of a drop of blood which is in the egg; and that the heart, together with the rest [of the parts] all sprout [165] simultaneously, as [occurs] in an ear of corn, from an imperceptible size. Is there only a drop of blood in the auricles whence bestowing heat upon all parts, receiving from none, it is the citadel and domicile of the heat, the household shrine [166] of that edifice, fowntayn conduit hed." [167]

More than eleven years after the making of his lecture notes Harvey, at the age of fifty, published his treatise of 1628; and later, after keeping silence for more than twenty years, he published together the two Exercises addressed to Riolanus. During these twenty years and more the blood must have been rising and the heart declining, in Harvey's esteem, as ruling powers in the body; for at the end of that time more than thirty-two years after the jotting down of the statements and varied conjectures of his lecture notes, he formally throws over Aristotle's primacy of the heart, in a passage near the close of the second Exercise to Riolanus. Of this passage the following is a part. Referring to certain opinions, mainly Aristotelian, regarding the heart and blood, Harvey says: —

"To speak openly, I do not believe that those things are so in the sense commonly received; and my opinion is inclined in the direction aforesaid by much which is visible in the generation of the parts, but which is not convenient to set down here. Soon, perhaps, I shall make public things even more wonderful and destined to cast even greater light upon natural philosophy.

"For the present I will only say and set forth without demonstration — by good leave of the learned and with due respect to the ancients — that the heart, as the beginning, author, source, and origin of everything in the body and the first cause of life, should be held to include the veins and all the arteries and also the contained blood; just as the brain, including all its nerves and sensory organs and spinal marrow, is the one adequate organ of sensation, as the phrase is. If by the word 'heart,' however, only the body of the heart be meant with its ventricles and auricles, I do not believe that it is the manufacturer of the blood; nor that the blood possesses vigor, faculty, reason,[168] motion, or heat, as the gift of the heart." [169]

In the second year after that of the Exercises to Riolanus Harvey's final publication, his treatise On Generation with appended essays, was given to the world, not long before his seventy-third birthday. During how many years this work had been in preparation we do not know; but it is avowedly based upon the views of Aristotle, whom Harvey styles his "*dux*" — his leader — as regards the subject of this treatise.[170] In it, to be sure, the ancient master is often weighed in the balance and found wanting by Harvey, who even questions whether Aristotle had seen for himself what he "narrates as to the generation of the chick," or "had accepted it from some expert." [171]   Nevertheless, it is with the doctrines of Aristotle that Harvey incessantly compares the results of observation.   Here the veteran records anew his denial of the Aristotelian primacy of the heart, and records as well his final emphatic assertion of the primacy of the blood.   In regard to these matters it is interesting to note the various grades of expression which appear to mirror in this single work the various phases of Harvey's thought.

In the following florid passage doubt of the primacy of the heart seems hardly even hinted at. Harvey says : —

"Certain of the parts themselves are said to be generative, such as the heart, from which Aristotle declares that the rest of the parts derive their origin; as is also clear from the history which I have given. The heart, I say — or at least its first beginning, to wit, the vesicle and leaping point — constructs the rest of the body to be its future abode; enters this when once built up, and hides in it, vivifies and governs it; fortifies it with ribs and sternum superimposed as a bulwark; and is a kind of household shrine, as it were, the first seat of the soul, the first receptacle and perennial soul-endowed [172] hearth of the innate heat, the source and origin of all the faculties, and their sole relief in calamity." [173]

Divergence from Aristotle in the matter of the heart is plainly marked, however, in the following passage of the same treatise, where Harvey says : —

"We find the blood formed before anything else in the egg and in the product of conception; [174] and almost at the same time the receptacles of the blood, the veins and the pulsating vesicle, become plainly visible. Wherefore, if the leaping point together with the veins and blood, which are all conspicuous as one single organ at the first beginning of the embryo, be accepted as the heart (the parenchyma of which is superadded to the vesicle later in the formation of the embryo), it is manifest that, accepted in this sense, that is, as an organ composed of parenchyma, ventricles, auricles, and blood, the heart in animals is in very truth, as Aristotle would have it, the principal and first generated part of the body; of which part, however, the first and foremost part is the blood, both by nature and in the order of generation." [175]

In the following third passage of the same treatise no reconciling interpretations of the master's words are to be found; flat disagreement with Aristotle is declared; and the "Sun of the Microcosm" [176] declines nearly to its simple modern status of a living pump! Harvey says : —

"Nor can I agree with Aristotle himself, who maintained that the heart is the primary generative part and that it is endowed with soul; for, truly, I believe the blood alone to be entitled to these distinctions, since the blood it is which first appears in generation; and that such is the case not only in the egg but also in every fœtus and very early animal embryo, shall at once be made plain.[177]

"At the beginning, I say, there appear the red leaping point, the pulsating vesicle, and filaments, derived thence, which contain blood in their interior. And, so far as can be discerned by accurate inspection, the blood is made before the leaping point is formed, and the blood is endowed with vital heat before it is set in motion by pulsation; and, further, as pulsation is begun in and by the blood, so at last it ends in the blood at the final instant of death. Indeed, by numerous experiments done upon the egg and otherwise I have made sure that it is the blood in which the power of returning to life persists, so long as the vital heat has not wholly vanished. And since the pulsating vesicle and the sanguineous filaments derived from it are seen before anything else, it stands to reason in my belief that the blood is prior to its receptacles — the contained, that is, to its container — since the latter is made for the use of the former. Therefore, it is probable that the filaments and the veins and then the vesicle and at length the heart, having organs destined to receive and retain the blood, are made for the sole purpose of transmitting and distributing it, and that the blood is the principal part of the body. . . .

"Therefore, relying with certainty upon what I have observed in the egg and in the dissection of living animals, I maintain against Aristotle that the blood is the primary generative part; and that the heart is its organ, destined to send it on a circuit. Surely the function of the heart is the propulsion of the blood, as is admirably clear in all animals that have blood; and in the generation of the chick the same duty falls to the pulsating vesicle, which in the very early embryos of animals [178] no less than in the egg I have often exhibited to view as something more minute than a spark, beating and when in action contracting itself and at the same time pressing out the blood contained in it, and in its relaxation receiving the same afresh." [179]

Whether in studying the foregoing passages we read Harvey's earlier jottings in his private note-book or the

deliberate statements published in his old age, it is
evident that to his mind the question of the primacy
of the blood versus the primacy of the heart depends
for answer upon the further question whether in the
development of the embryo the blood be made before
the heart, or the heart before the blood. In no other
part than one of these two can the primacy inhere, for
him; and whichever of these two has the priority
must be, to Harvey's mind, the origin of the other and
of the remaining parts and must continue to be the
"principal part" of the body throughout life. The
matter of the primacy thus resolves itself into one of
well-devised and accurate observation; and the discoverer is once more upon the ground where his undying
laurels grew. He, therefore, deals no longer "without
demonstration," as in the second Exercise to Riolanus,
but makes report of actual observations and so gives
ocular evidence in support of his views, remembering,
it may be, that he had said to Riolanus: "Soon, perhaps, I shall make public things even more wonderful
and destined to cast even greater light on natural
philosophy." [180] Harvey's contemporary Milton said
to Parliament: "Truth is compar'd in Scripture to a
streaming fountain; if her waters flow not in a per-
petuall progression, they sick'n into a muddy pool of
conformity and tradition." [181] These words seem timely
as we note the great discoverer, magnifying glass in hand,
searching in incubated eggs for an answer to the question, now wholly obsolete, whether the primacy of the
heart should not give way to the primacy of the blood.

"Surely," says Harvey, "this investigation is one of great
moment, to wit: whether or no the blood be present before the

pulse; and is the point [182] derived from the veins or the veins from
the point? So far as I have been able to observe, the blood appears
to exist before the pulse; and I will show cause for this opinion
as follows: On a Wednesday evening I put three eggs under a hen;
and having come back on the Saturday, a little before the same hour,
I found these eggs cold as though deserted by the hen. I opened
one of them, nevertheless, and came upon the beginning of a chick,
namely, a red sanguineous line at the circumference,[183] but at the
centre instead of the leaping point a point which was white and
bloodless. By this sign I perceived that the hen had left off sitting
not long before. So I caught her, shut her up in a box, and kept
her there the entire night; that is, after I had put under her the
two remaining eggs together with other fresh ones. What was the
result? Next day in the very early morning both eggs had revived;
and at the centre the beating point itself was visible, much smaller
than the white point; out of which, that is, out of the white one, it
made its appearance in diastole only, like a spark leaping forth
from a cloud: so that the red point seemed to me to flash out of
the white point; the leaping point being generated in the latter,
in one way or another; and the blood to be already in existence,
when the leaping point is brought into existence or at least into
motion. Indeed, I have very often found that even when the
leaping point lies still and devoid of all motion as though quite
dead, it recovers motion and pulsation again if warmed afresh.
From the foregoing I judge that in the order of generation the
point and the blood come into existence first; but that pulsation
does not come on till afterward. Certainly this is settled, viz.:
that of the future embryo nothing at all appears on this day [184]
except the sanguineous lines and the leaping point and also those
veins which grow all from one trunk (as this grows from the leaping
point) and are dispersed throughout the entire colliquative [185]
region in very many ramified filaments. . . .

"Toward the end of the fourth day and the beginning of the
fifth the sanguineous point is already increased in size and is seen
to be turned into a small and very delicate vesicle containing blood
within itself; which blood it drives out at every contraction, and
receives afresh when its diastole takes place.

"Up to this stage I have found it impossible to discriminate between the vessels; for the arteries are not to be distinguished from the veins either by their coats or by the pulse; and so I think it best to style all the vessels, indiscriminately, veins or, with Aristotle,[186] venous canals.[187] . . .

"On the sixth day . . . the parenchyma of the heart grows on to the pulsating vesicle; and shortly afterward the rudiments of the liver and of the lungs are discernible." [188]

It is clear that Harvey's hens did not very often take such well-timed steps against Aristotle; for in another passage of his treatise on generation, in summing up its events and their order, he frankly states the difficulties which render uncertain the question of priority between the blood and the heart. He speaks of "the first generated and generative part; that is to say, the blood together with its receptacles or, if your prefer, the heart with its veins." [189]   A few lines further on he says : —

"In the generation of this first part (which is accomplished in the egg on the fourth day) although I have not been able to observe any order, because all portions of the part aforesaid (namely, the blood, the veins and the pulsating vesicle) appear at the same time; nevertheless, my belief would be, as I have said, that the blood is present before the pulse; and that, therefore, in obedience to a law of nature the blood is prior to its receptacles, that is, to the veins." [190]

In Harvey's first publication, of 1628, we have read : —

"If you turn to the formation of the chick in the egg, the first thing to exist therein, as I have said, is a mere vesicle, or auricle, or pulsating drop of blood. Afterward, when growth has gone on, the heart is completed." [191]

In his last publication, of 1651, we have read : —

"So far as can be discerned by accurate inspection, the blood is made before the leaping point is formed, and the blood is endowed with vital heat before it is set in motion by pulsation; and further, as pulsation is begun in and by the blood, so at last it ends in the blood at the final instant of death." [192]

Harvey's own words in the foregoing two passages effectively sum up both the nature of his doctrine that the blood is the first part of the body to live, and the nature of his evidence. But the words of the second passage foreshadow a closely related doctrine, advanced and held by him on the evidence of observation, viz.: that the blood, being the first part to live, is also the last part of the body to die. That the first part to live is always the last to die, is a doctrine set forth by Aristotle. This, Harvey seems to accept without question and to apply upon proper evidence to the blood; as he accepts and warmly upholds the ancient master's doctrine that there is a primacy of the body. The results of observation have forced Harvey to transfer this primacy from the heart to the blood, but it is the Aristotelian primacy still. Presently he shall show us that the blood is not only the first part to live, but the last to die. Before he does so, however, let Aristotle speak for himself, saying briefly: —

"The point [193] of origin [of the rest of the body] is the first thing generated. The point of origin in the animals which possess blood is the heart; in the rest, the analogue thereof, as I have often said. Moreover, the fact that the heart is the first thing generated is evident, not only to the senses, but from its death.[194] For therein life ceases the last; and in all cases the last generated is the first to make an end, the first generated, the last to make an end; nature, as it were, doubling back and returning upon her point of origin whence she came.[195] For generation is the change from not being to being; destruction is the reverse change, from being to not being." [196]

Aristotle does not tell us why "in all cases . . . the first generated" is "the last to make an end," and *vice versa*. Let it suffice that Harvey accepts this sweeping doctrine. Now let him complete his evidence in favor of the primacy of the blood by showing that the blood is not only the first part to live and to live tenaciously, but the last part to die.

In a passage of the treatise On the Motion of the Heart and Blood, we have already read Harvey's promise to publish observations

"on the formation of the fœtus, where numerous problems of the following order can find a place: Why should this part be made or perfected earlier, that later? As regards the dominance of the members: Which part is the cause of the other? There are very many problems connected with the heart, such as: Why should it be the first thing (as Aristotle says in his third book On the Parts of Animals) [127] to acquire consistency, and be seen possessed of life, motion, and sensation, before anything has been perfected in the rest of the body? And in like manner regarding the blood: Why is it before all, and how possessed of the beginnings [128] of life and of the animal, and of the craving to move and be impelled hither and thither, to which end the heart would seem to have been made?" [129]

That Harvey should have printed this passage in 1628, in the same work with his repeated eulogies of the Aristotelian heart, shows that the idea of the possible primacy of the blood must have been in his mind early. It was, indeed, so from the jotting down of his private notes of 1616, to the publication of the Exercises to Riolanus in 1649 and the treatise On Generation in 1651. The same mental attitude is revealed, perhaps more strongly, in the following passage of an earlier chapter of Harvey's treatise of 1628. Here we come upon the thought that it may be the blood, and neither ventricle nor auricle, which is the last to die. Harvey says : —

"Besides this, however, I have occasionally observed, after the heart and even its right auricle [197] had ceased their pulsations as though in the act of dying, that an obscure motion and flow and a sort of palpitation manifestly remained in the blood itself contained in the right auricle, so long, that is, as the blood appeared to be imbued with heat and spirits. Something of the sort is very plainly to be seen at the beginning of the generation of an animal, in the hen's egg within the first seven days of incubation. There is present, first and before all else, a drop of blood which palpitates (as Aristotle also noted) ; from which, when growth has taken place and the chick has been formed to some extent, the auricles of the heart are made ; and in these, which pulsate perpetually, life inheres. . . .

"Whoever, therefore, shall choose to investigate more closely will say that the heart is not the first to live and the last to die, but that the auricles, and the part which answers thereto in serpents, fishes, and such animals, are alive sooner than the heart itself and also die later than the heart. Whether even earlier the blood itself, or the spirit, have not an obscure palpitation of its own, which it has seemed to me to retain after death, may well be questioned ; and whether we should not speak of life as beginning with palpitation." [198]

It is plain that fibrillar contractions of cardiac muscle misled Harvey into thinking and writing of "an obscure motion and flow," of "an obscure palpitation," of the blood itself within the dying auricle. It is plain that when he wrote his most famous treatise he was loath, even under Aristotle's leadership, to reach out so far beyond the evidence of the senses as to attribute the palpitation of the visible drop of blood in the very early embryo to anything but the hot blood itself. Later, in his treatise On Generation, he published a passage which in some ways runs parallel with the foregoing. In the earlier passage the results of observation are brought forward as food for thought; in the later one, as proofs of a theory, fully, clearly, and emphatically stated by a thinker who is near the end of life and is imparting his final judgment. This later passage is as follows: —

"In whatsoever part of the body heat and motion have their beginning, in that same part life also first arises and therein is extinguished last; nor may it be doubted that there, too, life has its innermost home, that there the soul itself has fixed its seat.

"The life then inheres in the blood (as we read also in Holy Writ [199]), because therein the life and the soul are manifest first and fail last. For, as I have said, in the dissection of living animals I have found repeatedly that, though the animal be dying and breathe no longer, nevertheless, the heart pulsates for some time and keeps the life in it. Moreover, when the heart is quieted you may see movement surviving in the auricles, and latest in the right auricle; and at length all pulsation ceasing there, you may find in the blood itself a kind of undulation and obscure agitation or palpitation, the last indication of life. And anyone can perceive that the blood retains in itself to the last the heat which is the author of pulsation and life; if this heat is once wholly extinguished and the blood now is blood no more, but cruor, so there is left no hope of a return to life again. Nevertheless, after all pulsation has disappeared, both in the egg, as I have said, and in dying animals, if you will make a gentle warm application, in the former case to the leaping point, in the latter to the right auricle of the heart, you shall see movement, pulsation, and life, renewed immediately by the blood; provided it have not utterly lost all its innate heat and vital spirits." [200]

How readily heat from without can revive the cool leaping point, is strikingly set forth by Harvey in another chapter of this treatise On Generation. He says: —

"Moreover, if an egg be exposed too long to a colder atmosphere, its leaping point pulsates less often and stirs more languidly; but if a warm finger be applied to it, or any other bland source of warmth, straightway it recovers strength and vigor. Indeed, when such a point has become gradually weak and though full of blood ceases to move at all and gives no sign of life, seeming utterly to have succumbed to death, if my lukewarm finger be placed over it for the space of twenty pulsations of my artery, behold! the little heart revives once more, becomes erect, and renews its pristine dance as though come back from Hades. This I myself and others, too, have brought about again and again by means of gentle warmth of any kind, such as that of a fire or of tepid water; thus at our pleasure being able to give over the poor little soul to death, or call it back to the light." [201]

As in the embryo the leaping point may be revived by external warmth, so may the heart in the full-grown bird. In his treatise of 1628 Harvey says:—

"In the pigeon, at any rate, at an actual experiment, after the heart had wholly ceased to move and even the auricles had left off moving, I placed my finger, wetted with saliva and warm, upon the heart and kept it there for a while; as the result of which fomentation the heart, as though restored to strength and life again, and its auricles with it, were seen to move and contract and relax themselves and, as it were, to be recalled from death." [202]

In his treatise On Generation, Harvey confirms the doctrine of the primacy of the blood by citing observations made upon sluggish or hibernating animals and also certain morbid phenomena in man, as follows:—

"This, too, clearly follows from many observations; especially the cases of certain animals which possess blood yet live a long time without a pulse; and of some which lie hidden the whole winter and, nevertheless, continue alive, although meanwhile all movement of the heart has ceased and their lungs enjoy a rest from breathing, like people who lie half dead and pulseless in syncope or faintness or hysterical affections." [203]

So Harvey convinced himself, by observation, that the first part of the developing embryo to appear is the blood of the "sanguineous lines"; after this the blood which seems to palpitate of itself at the leaping point, which later develops into a pulsating vesicle wherein blood is contained within a contractile wall; to this being superadded still later the contractile parenchyma of the heart.   Also, by observation, he convinced himself that in a dying animal the blood within the right auricle may palpitate of itself after the palpitations due to contractions of the auricular wall have ceased. Thus was Harvey led to believe that the blood and not the heart is the first part to live and the last to die, the principal part of the body, the generator of the heart and of all the rest.   In spite of his appeal to observation, his impressive primacy of the blood is now as completely forgotten in its turn as is Aristotle's impressive primacy of the heart, which Harvey felt called upon to supersede.   Naturally in this matter the great discoverer used true methods of investigation; and doubtless his imperfect conclusions were due in large part to the weakness of his magnifying glasses and to the deficient technique of his day.   Harvey said of himself, speaking generally, that he trusted much to the plain use of his senses.[204]   That he did so, was well for him and for all mankind; yet because of this very trust he did not always escape the pitfalls dug by what we now call "naked-eye" appearances.

CHAPTER VII

THE CAUSE OF THE HEART-BEAT

THE primacy of the blood was no isolated fact for Harvey, but one linked with the very existence of the circulation. This primacy depended largely upon the blood being the primal abode of the innate heat. Palpitation produced by the innate heat in the blood itself, he held to be the first sign of life in the embryo and the last sign of life in the dying creature; and a swelling produced by the innate heat, he held to take place throughout life, localized in the blood just outside of the entrance to the heart. This local swelling of the blood was, to him, the exciting cause of the heart-beat and, therefore, of the circulation. We have heard him deny that the blood possesses motion "as the gift of the heart." [205] We can now grasp the probable meaning of this denial. He would not have been illogical had he said also that the heart possesses motion as the gift of the blood. This view of the cause of the heart-beat was first set forth by Harvey in 1649 in the Exercises to Riolanus, and in immediate connection with declarations in favor of the primacy of the blood, which also was first formally advocated in those Exercises. As we know, the question of this primacy had given Harvey food for thought long before. But his view of the cause of the heart-beat is not to be found in his lecture notes, nor in the treatise of 1628, and may well have been a later outgrowth from the larger doctrine of the primacy of the blood.

Let us now turn to the Exercises and to Harvey's own account of the cause of the heart-beat. The first passage to be quoted begins with a few sentences which have been introduced previously, but which form a necessary cue for the statement we are to study. Harvey says to Riolanus : —

"For the present I will only say and set forth without demonstration — by good leave of the learned and with due respect to the ancients — that the heart, as the beginning, author, source, and origin of everything in the body and the first cause of life, should be held to include the veins and all the arteries and also the contained blood; just as the brain, including all its nerves and sensory organs and spinal marrow, is the one adequate organ of sensation, as the phrase is. If by the word 'heart,' however, only the body of the heart be meant with its ventricles and auricles, I do not believe that it is the manufacturer of the blood; nor that the blood possesses vigor, faculty, reason,[168] motion, or heat, as the gift of the heart. Moreover, I judge the cause of diastole and expansion not to be the same as that of systole and contraction, either in the arteries, or in the auricles or the ventricles of the heart; but that part of the pulse which is called diastole has another cause, different from the systole, and always and everywhere must precede every systole; I judge the first cause of expansion to be the innate heat and expansion to occur first in the blood itself, gradually thinned and swelling up like matters in fermentation, and to be extinguished last in the same; and I accept Aristotle's parallel with pottage or milk with this proviso, that the rising or falling of the blood is not brought about by vapors, or exhalations, or spirits, excited into some vaporous or aërial form, and is caused, not by an external agent, but by an internal principle, and is regulated by nature.

"Nor is the heart (like a hot kettle), as some imagine, the origin of the heat and of the blood in the same sense as a hot coal or a fireplace. The blood rather imparts heat to the heart, as to all other parts, than receives heat from it, for the blood is, of all things within the body, the hottest; and so the heart is provided with coronary arteries and veins for the same purpose as that of the arteries and veins of other parts, viz.: to secure an influx of heat which shall foster and preserve. Hence it is to use convertible terms to say that all the hotter parts contain more blood and that the richer they are in blood, the hotter they are. It is in this sense that the heart, so remarkable for its cavities, should be reckoned a workshop, source, perpetual fire-place; it is like a hot kettle by virtue, not of its body, but of its contained blood, in the same sense in which the liver, the spleen, the lungs, and other parts are reckoned hot; because they contain many veins or vessels containing blood. In this way also I maintain that the native heat, or innate warmth, being the common instrument of all the functions, is likewise the prime efficient cause of the pulse. This I do not now assert positively, but only propose as a thesis. Whatever may be brought forward to the contrary by learned and upright men without scurrilous language, clamor, or contumely, I shall be glad to know, and whoever shall do that will earn my gratitude." [206]

Harvey has thus transferred to the blood the primacy of the body, making the blood in place of the Aristotelian heart the primal abode of the innate heat, "the common instrument of all the functions." Nevertheless, the blood of the Harveian circulation cannot perform the duties of the primacy without the aid of Aristotle.

If we turn from the Exercises to the treatise On Generation, published about two years later, we find the author saying: —

"The primacy of the blood is evident from this also, that the pulse has its origin in the blood. For since a pulsation consists of two parts, to wit: an expansion and a contraction, or a diastole and systole, and since the prior of these movements is the expansion, it is plain that this action is due to the blood, but that the contraction is set a-going in the egg by the pulsating vesicle, as by the heart in the chick, by means of its own fibres as though by an instrument devised for that purpose.   It is certain also that the aforesaid vesicle and, at a later time, the cardiac auricle from which pulsation starts, is excited by the blood, which expands to the motion which constricts.   The diastole, I say, is produced by the blood which swells up as if with interior spirits; and so Aristotle's opinion as to the heart's pulsation — namely, that it is produced after the manner of ebullition — is in some measure true.   For the same thing which we see every day in milk heated over the fire and in the fermentation of our beer, comes into play also in the pulsation of the heart, in which the blood swells as from some fermentation, is expanded, and subsides; and what is brought about in the cases aforesaid by accident and by an external agent, to wit, by adventitious heat from somewhere, is effected in the blood by the internal heat or innate spirits, and is also regulated by the soul in conformity to nature, and is kept up for the health of living things.   Pulsation, therefore, is accomplished by a double agency: that is to say, the expansion or dilatation is accomplished by the blood, but the contraction or systole is accomplished in the egg by the membrane of the vesicle, in the fœtus after birth by the auricles and ventricles of the heart; and these alternate and mutually associated efforts once begun, the blood is impelled through the whole body, and thus the life of animals is perpetuated." [207]

Nearly two thousand years before Harvey's time Aristotle had said : —

"The volume of leaven [208] changes from small to great, by its more solid part becoming liquefied and its liquid, vaporized.[209] This is brought about in animals by the nature of the psychical heat, but in the case of leaven by the heat of the blended juices." [210]

Moreover, Aristotle, as Harvey says, had likened to "ebullition" [211] what Aristotle himself described as "the pulsation which occurs at the heart, at which the heart is always to be seen incessantly at work." "For," says Aristotle, "ebullition takes place when liquid is vaporized [212] by heat; for it rises up owing to its bulk becoming greater." [213]   He continues : —

"In the heart the swelling up from heat of the liquid which is always arriving from the food produces pulsation, for the swelling rises against the outer tunic [214] of the heart; and this process is always and incessantly going on, for the liquid is always and incessantly flowing in, out of which the nature of the blood arises; for the blood is first worked up in the heart.   The thing is plain in generation from the beginning; for before the vessels have been marked out the heart is to be seen containing blood.   Hence, too, it pulsates more in the young than in the old; for the vapor [215] arises more abundantly in the young.

"All the vessels also pulsate and do so simultaneously one with another, because they are dependent upon the heart.[216]   This is always moving, so that they, too, are always moving, and simultaneously one with another, when [217] the heart moves.   Leaping [of the heart], [218] then, is the reaction which takes place against the condensation produced by cold, and pulsation is the vaporization [219] of heated liquid." [220]

In another treatise Aristotle says: "In all animals the blood pulsates in the vessels everywhere at the same time." [221]   It is interesting, in a negative way, that his sweeping and faulty references to the pulsation of the vessels put into words no physiological idea except the vague one of "dependence" on the heart.

One may be tempted to see in the seething of the heart's blood the source of some of those spirits within the body elsewhere than in and about the heart, of which one gets brief ill-defined glimpses here and there in the genuine works of Aristotle.   But no words of his can be adduced to confirm such a conjecture.

Evidently, however, the seething of the nascent blood suffices, in Aristotle's eyes, to explain both the phases of the heart-beat; for both the rising and the falling of the wall of the hot central laboratory of the

blood are movements as passive apparently as those
of the lid of a boiling pot. One may be excused for
wondering at the crudity of such a conception; nor
is one's wonder lessened by recalling that elsewhere
in Aristotle's works he places at the heart the central
origin of the bodily movements. But when it is recalled, as well, that Aristotle was totally ignorant of the
function of muscle and, therefore, even of the mode of
working of the limbs, his doctrine of the heart-beat may
seem less amazing.

There are indications that the function of muscle,
though unknown to Aristotle, was known not long
after his time,[222] and in Galen's time that function was
entirely familiar, he styling the muscles "the organs of
voluntary movement," and calling their contraction
their "systole," a term which has survived only in
connection with the heart and arteries.[223] For Harvey,
born more than thirteen centuries after Galen's death,
the function of muscle was a portion of ancient knowledge; and in his treatise On the Motion of the Heart
and Blood, he expressly states that the heart, including the auricles, is muscular both in structure and in
function. The opinions of Harvey's day rendered
these statements by no means superfluous.[224] Naturally, therefore, in accepting the aid of the Aristotelian
seething of the blood in connection with the heart-
beat Harvey utilized only the force of expansion thus
generated, and obtained from muscle the force of
contraction which he required. Indeed, the conception of the auricles and ventricles as muscular force-
pumps was fundamental to his doctrine of the circulation. Moreover, we have found Harvey careful to

limit and mitigate the expansion of the blood, he saying to Riolanus : —

"I accept Aristotle's parallel with pottage or milk with this proviso, that the rising or falling of the blood is not brought about by vapors, or exhalations, or spirits, excited into some vaporous or aërial form, and is caused, not by an external agent, but by an internal principle, and is regulated by nature." [224]

Long before, indeed, he had jotted down a terse statement among his lecture notes which is fatal to any extreme development of the Aristotelian idea. In dealing with the action of the heart he had written : —

"To what end?   Aristotle : To none, but a passive process, as in boiling pottage.   But when wounded it gives out not wind, but blood." [226]

Harvey, therefore, could do no less than criticize adversely his famous contemporary, the philosopher Descartes, for accepting in its entirety Aristotle's doctrine of the heart-beat.   Referring to Descartes he says : —

"Nor in the matter of the pulse am I satisfied with the efficient cause thereof which he, following Aristotle, has laid down as the same at the systole as at the diastole, to wit : an effervescence of the blood like that produced in boiling.   For the movements aforesaid are sudden strokes and swift beats ; while in fermentation or ebullition nothing rises up and collapses thus, as it were in the twinkling of an eye, but there is a slow swelling with a sufficient subsidence.   By means of dissection, moreover, one can discern for oneself that the ventricles of the heart are expanded as well as filled by the constriction of the auricles and are increased in size proportionately, according as they are filled more or less ; and that the expansion of the heart is a movement of a certain violence, produced by impulsion, not by attraction [227] of some sort." [228]

In a letter written four years after the publication of
the Exercises to Riolanus and two years after that of
the treatise On Generation, Harvey sets forth anew,
with admirable clearness and brevity, his doctrine as
to the nature and cause of the systole of the ventricles.
In this he stands upon purely modern ground as an
observer, and his words are free from all Aristotelian
tinge.   Referring to another physiologist he says : —

"I could wish, however, that he had observed this one thing,
namely, that the motion which the heart enjoys is of a threefold
kind, to wit: a systole, in which the heart contracts itself and
drives out the blood contained in it ; and then a certain relaxation,
of a character contrary to the foregoing motion, a relaxation in
which the fibres of the heart which make for motion are slackened.
The two motions aforesaid are inherent in the very substance of the
heart, just as in all other muscles.   Finally, there takes place a
diastole, in which the heart is expanded by blood impelled into its
ventricles out of the auricles ; and the heart is incited to its own
contraction by this filling and expansion of the ventricles ; and the
motion aforesaid always precedes the systole, which follows at
once." [229]

Harvey materially clarifies his doctrine of the nature
and cause of the heart-beat in the following admirable
summary.   In the second Exercise to Riolanus he
says : —

"Since I see that many are embarrassed and doubt the circulation, and that some attack it, because they have not understood
me thoroughly ; for their sake I will recapitulate briefly what I
meant to say in my little book on the motion of the heart and blood.
The blood contained in the veins, where its deeps are, as it were,
where it is most abundant, that is, in the vena cava close to the base
of the heart and to the right auricle, gradually grows warm and thin
by reason of its own internal heat, and swells and rises up like
matters in fermentation ; whereby the auricle is dilated, contracts

itself by reason of its own pulsific faculty, and propels the blood
promptly and frequently into the right ventricle of the heart. This,
when filled, frees itself of blood at its succeeding systole by the
impulsion thereof and, as the tricuspid valve is a bar to the egress
of the blood, drives it where an open door is offered, into the arterial
vein, and thereby brings about the expansion of the latter. The
blood within the arterial vessels cannot now go back in opposition
to the sigmoid valve, while at the same time the lungs are widened
and enlarged and then narrowed by inspiration and expiration —
and with the lungs their vessels also — and offer to the blood aforesaid a path and transit into the venous artery. The left auricle
accomplishes its movement, its rhythm, its order [of events], its
function, at the same time and in the same way as the right auricle,
and in like manner sends on into the left ventricle out of the vessels
aforesaid the same blood which the right auricle had sent on into
the right ventricle. As a result the left ventricle, at the same time
and in the same way as the right, impels the blood into the cavity
of the aorta and consequently into all the branches of the artery,
the return of the blood whence it had come being prevented in the
same way as before by the barrier of an opposing valve. The
arteries are filled by this sudden impulsion and, as they cannot
unload themselves as suddenly, are expanded, receive an impulse,
and undergo their diastole." [230]

Harvey seems to have attributed more importance
to the auricular systoles than do the physiologists of
to-day, he making the ventricles depend very greatly
for their charge of blood upon the systole of the auricles. This view appears in three passages already
quoted; and is tersely put by Harvey when he says
elsewhere that the heart "is dilated by the auricle,
contracts of itself"; [231] that "the auricles are prime
movers of the blood." [232] The unduly high value set
by him upon the auricular systole agrees well with the
polemical vigor with which Harvey exalted impulsion
and rejected suction,[233] in his general physiology as

well as in the physiology of the heart. In the heart especially the force of suction had played for centuries a part which Harvey rejected more completely than the physiologists of to-day feel warranted in doing. Again he shall speak for himself, saying tersely : —

"Hence it is made plain how the blood enters the ventricles; not by reason of being drawn in, or of the heart expanding, but because sent in by the pulse of the auricles." [234]

"The expansion of the heart," he has told us already, "is a movement of a certain violence, produced by impulsion, not by attraction of some sort." He says that he maintains these views

"against the commonly received opinion; because neither the heart nor anything else can so expand itself that it can draw anything into itself in its diastole, unless as a sponge does which has first been forcibly compressed and is returning to its natural state." [235]

But, one may ask oneself, how does that modified seething in the vena cava which produces the diastole of the right auricle produce the diastole, the simultaneous diastole, of the left auricle? In his lecture notes Harvey had stated, as Columbus had before him, that the venous artery does not pulsate — at least, he means, not in the same sense as the auricle, or ventricle, or artery. [236] Obviously regarding the left auricle there could be available, for Harvey, no explanation parallel to that of to-day, viz. : the swift conduction of a stimulus from point to point of the texture of a wall which is common to both auricles. He is careful to state that corresponding auricular events occur simultaneously and in the same way in the two auricles; and incidentally but frankly he confesses ignorance of the reasons why, in the following passage : —

"From those who declare the causes and reasons of all things in such a smattering way, I would be glad to learn how it is that both eyes move together hither and thither and in every direction when they look; how it is that this eye does not turn by itself in that direction, that eye in this; likewise, both auricles of the heart; and so forth." [237]

The circulation of the blood, then, according to the final view of its discoverer, is maintained by a self-regulating mechanism worked by causes operating within the blood itself, the "principal part" of the body. The systolic muscular contractions of the walls of the ventricles are caused by direct mechanical stimulation (in modern language) due to diastolic distension by blood of the relaxed muscular walls of these chambers. The blood which distends the ventricles is driven forcibly into them by the auricular systole, the muscular walls of the auricles having been stimulated to contract by diastolic distention due likewise to blood.

So much of Harvey's doctrine of the heart-beat, although not that of to-day, is very effective as physiology, and has advanced with modern swiftness far beyond that of his predecessors. It seems strange, therefore, even to one familiar with the movement of the Renaissance, to be swept back nearly two thousand years under Harvey's guidance to reach the underlying cause of the phenomena. According to him the distention which stimulates the right auricle to contract is produced by an expansion of the blood of the great veins, due to the innate heat. The Harveian heart-beat is caused and initiated by an Aristotelian swelling up of the hot blood. Both this expansion and the fiery central hearth at which it is produced have been expelled by Harvey from within the fully developed heart; and the primal abode of the innate heat has been transferred to the blood, with which that heat has been intimately incorporated by him. Just without the heart, moreover, Harvey has established anew the Aristotelian seething; making this the result of what we to-day may style a localized automatism of the conjoined heat and blood. He has localized this automatism of the hot blood "in the vena cava, close to the base of the heart and to the right auricle," *i.e.*, close to that region at and between the mouths of the two venæ cavæ of our present terminology, where the physiology of to-day places, not within the blood but in the texture of the walls which contain it, the seat of what is prepotent in determining the rhythm of the mammalian heart-beat.

Observation shows that from seemingly pulseless peripheral veins the blood continuously enters the venæ cavæ, which pulsate visibly in the region of Harvey's swelling of the blood. Yet in his lecture notes, in dealing with the significance of the thick resistent walls of the arterial vein and the aorta, he wrote: "Neither the vena cava nor the venous artery is of such construction, because they do not pulsate but, rather, are attracted." [238] On a neighboring page he had written: —

"At the same time [that] the pulse of the artery is perceived by touch, the vena cava is attracted, as it were." [239]

We will not now search for what he meant by saying that "the vena cava is attracted, as it were." Clearly, however, in denying that it pulsates, he meant not to deny that its wall moves rhythmically, but to deny only that this movement is of the nature of what he styles pulsation in the case of the auricles or the ventricles, or the arteries, or the arterial vein.

We know not what influence the rhythmic movements of the wall of the vena cava may have had upon Harvey's transfer to its cavity of the Aristotelian seething of the blood. To this was referable the palpitation seen by him in the blood itself as the first sign of life in the embryo and the last sign of life in the dying animal; and in this same familiar seething he found ready to his hand a life-long cause for the visible sharp expansion of the auricle in its diastole, for which expansion he could find no such obvious muscular cause as for the corresponding expansion of the ventricle or the arteries. The seething of the blood, however, was carefully kept by him below the point of vaporization and adapted to maintain the circulation by keeping the muscular cardiac pump at work.

Connected with Harvey's doctrine of the cause of the heart-beat there is a point which a student of his thought may find knotty, despite the aid of a well-developed historical sense. Harvey made the systolic contraction of auricle or ventricle dependent on the mechanical stimulus of its next preceding diastolic distension. It is not quite easy to see how he found this process compatible with the orderly recurrence of all the systolic contractions in the beating of a nearly empty heart. It is well known that the heart may beat for a while when cut out of the body, when, therefore, the heart is nearly drained of blood. In the treatise of 1628 Harvey himself speaks of studying the ventricular systole of "the heart of an eel, taken out and laid upon the table or the hand"; and says that the phenomena seen in this are seen likewise "in the hearts of little fishes, and in those colder animals in which the heart is conical or elongated."[240] In his lecture notes he says, we remember, that "the auricles pulsate after removal of the heart, because of the multitudinous blood."[241] But this jotting, written only as a brief reminder for himself, is obscure to others. By the word "heart" Harvey means sometimes the ventricular mass without the auricles and sometimes the ventricular mass and the auricles taken together. Hence it is uncertain whether the above reference be to auricles left attached to the body or removed with the ventricular mass. In neither case is it easy to imagine effective distention produced by the seething even of "the multitudinous blood." However, in the same lecture notes a few pages farther on Harvey says: "Nevertheless, the heart pulsates, cut away from the auricles;"[242] and in the treatise of 1628 he says:—

"The heart of the eel and of some fishes, and of animals even, when taken out, pulsates without auricles; indeed, if you cut it in pieces you shall see its divided parts contracting and relaxing separately; so that in these creatures the body of the heart pulsates and palpitates after the auricles have ceased to move. Is this, however, peculiar to the animals which are more tenacious of life, whose radical moisture is more glutinous, or rich, and sticky,[243] and not so readily dissolved? For in eels the thing is apparent even in their flesh, which retains the power of motion after they have been skinned, drawn, and cut in pieces."[244]

At this point we may recall the following words of our author : —

"I affirm also that in this way the native heat or innate warmth, being the common instrument of all the functions, is likewise the prime efficient cause of the pulse." [245]

Should we hazard the improbable guess that Harvey meant his cause of the heart-beat to be effective only in warm-blooded animals, we must remind ourselves that it certainly was well known to him as to all the other physicians of his day that the heart of the mammal beats after excision. If few had made experiments, all had studied Galen ; and Galen cites the beating of the heart after excision as evidence that its beat does not depend upon the nervous system, the context making it obvious that he refers to the heart-beat of the mammal. Moreover, he makes it evident that the striking phenomenon in question must have been seen by the ancients at the altar, as an incident of sacrificial rites.[246] This fact makes it easy to understand how it happened that earlier still, at least two centuries before Galen's time, the layman Cicero, one of Harvey's favorite authors, should have made a stoic say : —

"It has often been observed that, when the heart of some animal has been torn out, it palpitates with a mobility which imitates the swiftness of fire." [247]

Moreover, thirty-five years before Harvey was born, even the beating of the excised human heart had been seen by Vesalius, and referred to in his celebrated treatise on anatomy, as an incident of one of the barbarous executions of the sixteenth century.[248]

By no means in accord with the cause of the heart-beat first advocated by Harvey in 1649, is an experiment which he himself had brought forward in support of the circulation in 1628. In the famous treatise of that year he tells us that if the vena cava of a living snake be compressed at a point some distance away from the heart, the vein between that point and the heart is nearly emptied by the heart-beat, and the heart itself becomes paler and shrinks from lack of blood "and at length beats more languidly." [249] These words show that in this experiment the orderly heart-beats must have continued after the blood remaining in the vena cava had become too scanty to excite them by its expansion in accordance with his doctrine. It is, therefore, an interesting question how Harvey could reconcile the beating of the empty heart with his belief as to the "prime efficient cause" of its beat.

CHAPTER VIII

HARVEY'S DELINEATION OF THE VENOUS RETURN

IT may seem surprising that the discoverer of the venous return felt the need of a *deus ex machina* to distend the right auricle. On reflection, however, ought it to surprise us that, although we find the muscular power of the heart sufficient to complete the Harveian circulation, Harvey himself did not, but eked it out with Aristotelian forces? Vigorous as Harvey was, he could not make smooth the road which he himself had broken. For instance, he could not study, like ourselves, the return of the blood to the heart in the opened chest of an animal anæsthetized and curarized. The knowledge gained by his own tireless investigations did not suffice to teach him what we now know, viz.: that the unaided force of the systole of the left ventricle is sufficient to distend the right auricle with blood and to charge with blood the right ventricle as well.

The essence of Harvey's great discovery is his reversal of the immemorial direction of the venous flow, which he also proved to be abundant and rapid. But the laws which rule this flow were not, and could not be, patent to him as to us, owing to the imperfect physiological knowledge of his day. Hence at times his statements as to the movement of the blood are conceived in what, to borrow an architectural phrase, may be called a "transition style." As a sequel to his doctrine of the cause of the heart-beat let us pass in review some of these statements; but, first, let us briefly note a few facts which may help us to realize the imperfect state of the science of physics in Harvey's day.

Harvey was fourteen years younger than Galileo, who struck crippling blows at the Aristotelian physics, yet could not explain the common pump;[250] and Harvey's discovery of the circulation was made public thirteen years before the momentous work on the movement of liquids done by Torricelli, who was thirty years younger than Harvey.[250] Moreover, it was only a year before the publication of the Exercises to Riolanus in Harvey's old age that Blaise Pascal supplied the final proof that the mercurial column below the vacuum of Torricelli's barometer is really sustained by the pressure of the atmosphere.[250] It was not till one hundred years after the publication of Harvey's discovery that the Reverend Stephen Hales published the first comparative manometric measurements of the blood-pressure in the arteries and the veins of the same living animal, and stated in his preface that "the animal fluids move by Hydraulick and Hydrostatical Laws." [251]

Now let us turn to some delineations of the movement of the blood made by Harvey himself. I have found no evidence that he knew the venous flow to be promoted by the aspiration of the chest; but he knew well the effect of the muscular movements of the body upon that flow. Of course he had a perfect grasp of the fundamental truth that the main cause of the venous return is the forcible emptying of the ventricles into the arteries. He says to Riolanus : —

EXERCITATIO
ANATOMICA DE
MOTV CORDIS ET SAN-
GVINIS IN ANIMALI-
BVS,
GVILIELMI HARVEI ANGLI,
Medici Regii, & Professoris Anatomiæ in Col-
legio Medicorum Londinensi.

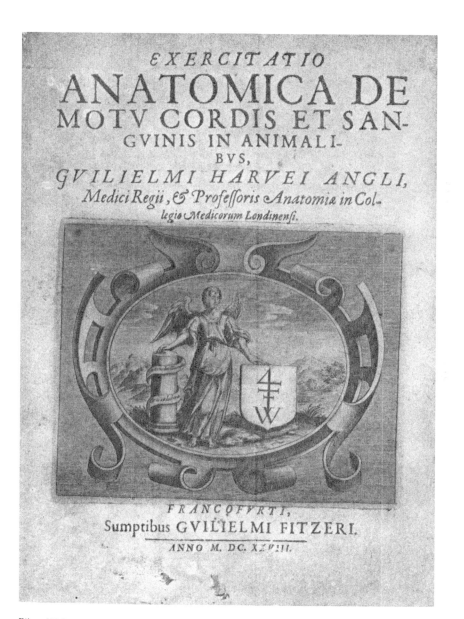

FRANCOFVRTI,
Sumptibus GVILIELMI FITZERI.
ANNO M. DC. XXVIII.

The Title-page of William Harvey's *Exercitatio Anatomica de Motu Cordis et Sanguinis in Animalibus*, Frankfort, 1628.

"Among these things should be noted the force and violence and rapid vehemence which we perceive by touch and sight in the heart and greater arteries; and the systole and diastole of the pulse in the larger and warmer animals I do not affirm to be the same in all the vessels which contain blood, nor in all blood-containing animals; but to be such and so ample in all that as a result thereof a streaming and an accelerated course of the blood through the small arteries, the porosities of the parts, and the branches of all the veins are necessarily brought about; and as a result thereof a circulation.[252] . . . In the case of the arteries, over and above the shock, pulse, or vibration of the blood (which is not equally perceptible in all), a continual flow and movement thence take place until the blood returns to the point whence it started first, namely, the right auricle." [253]

With the calm quantitative account which a reader of Hales' "Statical Essays" will find given by that clergyman of his epoch-making physical experiments upon the blood-pressure, it is interesting to compare the following vivid qualitative recital of inferences made from surgical observations by his great predecessor. Harvey says: —

"Moreover, whoever shall have seen and thought upon the amount of difficulty and exertion with which the blood is stanched by compression, ligatures, or various appliances, when it leaps impetuously out of a petty artery, even the smallest, which has been cut or torn in two; and shall have seen or thought upon the amount of force with which the blood, as though thrown out from a syringe, flings off and drives before it the whole of the appliances, or traverses them — that man will hardly believe it probable, I think, that any of the blood can pass backward against so great an impulse and influx of the entering blood, unless from a point whence it is driven back with equal force." [254]

Harvey rightly discountenanced the ancient idea of direct anastomoses between the mouths of veins and the mouths of arteries, as opposed to fine and

multiplied communications. In some situations, however, he admitted that ampler communications exist
comparable to such anastomoses; and it throws light
upon his state of mind as to the movement of the blood
that, despite his recognition of the very forcible exit
of the blood from the arteries, he suggested in his old
age that in the cases aforesaid regurgitation from vein
to artery is guarded against by a valvular arrangement,
the terminal part of the artery traversing the wall of
the vein obliquely, as the ureter traverses the wall of
the bladder and as the biliary duct traverses the wall
of the duodenum.[255] We should not forget that in his
day the capillary vessels, the existence of the corpuscles,
and the chemistry of the blood were still unknown; so
that the passage into the veins of the mysterious hot
vital liquid through the "porosities" of the parts
might naturally present itself to his mind in a way very
strange to us. He tells us this: —

"The blood does not take its course through the looser texture
of flesh and parenchyma in the same way as through the more com-
pact consistency of tendinous parts. Indeed, the thinner and purer
and more spirituous part passes through more quickly; the thicker,
more earthy, ill-composed [256] part tarries longer and is rejected." [257]

After more than twenty years of the comment and
criticism, called forth by his treatise of 1628, he said to
Riolanus: —

"As to whether the moving blood be attracted, or impelled, or
move itself by virtue of its own intrinsic nature, enough has been
said in my little book on the motion of the heart and blood." [258]

Yet about two years after the Exercises to Riolanus,
Harvey, in writing a private letter, judged it necessary

to accentuate, as follows, his denial that forces of
attraction really play the part in physiology which the
ancients had conceded to them. Speaking of the
impulsion of the blood through the arteries, he says : —

"Indeed, the passage of the blood into the veins is brought about
by that impulsion and not by any dilatation of the veins whereby,
like bellows, they draw in the blood." [259]

But, despite the foregoing utterances and other such,
his statements are sometimes vague and sometimes
quite unexpected, regarding the nature of the movement of the blood in the veins. Indeed, in 1628 he
speaks quite as a disciple of Aristotle. He says regarding the flow in the arteries : —

"For this distribution and movement of the blood there is need
of impetus and violence and of an impeller such as the heart. Partly
because the blood readily concentrates and gathers together of
itself — toward its seat of origin, as it were,[260] or as a part to the
whole, or as a drop of the water sprinkled upon a table to the mass
thereof — as the blood habitually and very speedily does from slight
causes, from cold, fear, horror, and other causes of this sort ; partly,
also, because the blood is pressed out of the capillary veins into the
small branches and thence into the greater by the movements of
the limbs and the compression of the muscles ; the blood is more
disposed and prone to move from the circumference on the center
than the other way, even supposing no valves to be present as a
hindrance. In order, therefore, to relinquish its seat of origin, and
enter constricted and colder places, and move in opposition to its
bent,[261] the blood has need not only of violence but of an impeller,
such as is the heart alone, and after the fashion described already."[262]

This picture of the blood hesitating to leave its warm
cardiac birthplace for the chill regions of the periphery,
but very ready to return, has a tone far from hydraulic,
but may so much the better prepare us for the view,

made public by Harvey in his old age, that the blood
is the primal seat of the soul itself.   Except in the light
of the foregoing passage the following words would
be quite obscure.   He says that the auricles

"are filled as being the storehouse and reservoir [263] of the blood,
the blood turning of itself and compressed toward the center by
the movement of the veins." [264]

With due allowance for the use of modes of expression no longer familiar we find Harvey in 1649 handling
the venous flow with no very modern touch, in the
following passage — a passage which also reminds us
that not till twelve years later, four years after Harvey's
death, did Malpighi announce his discovery of the
capillary blood-vessels in the lung of the frog. [265]   Harvey says to Riolanus : —

"The arteries are never depleted except into the veins or the
porosities of the parts, but are continually stuffed full by the pulse
of the heart; but in the vena cava and the circulatory vessels, into
which the blood glides at a quick pace and hastens toward the heart,
there would be the greatest scarcity of blood, did not all the parts
incessantly pour out again the blood poured into them.   Add,
also, that the impetus of the blood which is urged and driven at
every pulsation into all parts of the second and third regions, forces
the blood contained therein from the porosities into the little veins
and from the branches into the larger vessels; this being effected
also by the motion and compression of the surrounding parts;
for contents are squeezed out of whatever contains them, when it
is compressed and narrowed.   So by the movements of the muscles
and limbs the venous branches which creep on between are pressed
upon and narrowed, and push on the blood from the lesser toward
the greater." [266]

A similar touch of vagueness is perceptible when
the venous flow is dealt with by Harvey in that very

same résumé of the circulation which seats the underlying cause of the pulse in the hot blood of the vena cava
close to the auricle. In that résumé he says to Riolanus : —

"I assert, further, that the blood in the veins courses always
and everywhere from the lesser into the greater and hastens from
all parts toward the heart; whence I gather that the amount, continuously sent into the arteries, which the arteries have received
is transferred through the veins, and at length returns and flows
back whence it first was impelled; and that in this wise the blood
is moved in a circle in flux and reflux by the heart, by an impulsion
the impetus of which forces the blood through all the arterial filaments; and that afterward in a continuous flow from all parts it
goes back through the veins, one after another, by which it is absorbed, drained away, and transported." [267]

As to the flow in the lungs Harvey says in the treatise
of 1628 : —

"It being the will of nature that the blood itself be strained
through the lungs, she was obliged to superadd the right ventricle,
in order that by the beat thereof the blood might be driven through
the lungs themselves, out of the vena cava into the cavity of the
left ventricle." [268]

We have already found Harvey saying to Riolanus, in
regard to the pulmonary transit, that the blood within
the branches of the arterial vein

"cannot now go back in opposition to the sigmoid valve, while at
the same time the lungs are widened and enlarged and then narrowed, by inspiration and expiration, and with the lungs their vessels also, and offer to the blood aforesaid a path and transit into the
venous artery." [269]

More than thirty-two years earlier Harvey had written
in his note-book the following words : —

"N.B.   The lungs by their movement in subsiding propel blood from the arterial vein into the venous artery and thence into the left auricle." [270]

When we review and ponder the foregoing delineations of the character of the movement of the blood, we may cease to wonder that Harvey did not recognize the simple hydraulic cause of the distention of the right auricle and felt obliged to seek a more recondite explanation thereof, finding this in an Aristotelian expansion of the hot blood.

CHAPTER IX

No doctrine of Harvey sounds stranger to a biologist of to-day than his doctrine that the blood is the seat of the soul; nor does any other belief of the great discoverer reveal him more clearly to be a link between the old and the new; not simply an innovator who fixed a gulf between them. We have heard him explicitly deny in his old age the Aristotelian doctrine that the heart "is endowed with soul." We have seen that thirty-five years earlier he had jotted down in his note-book these words: "The soul is in the blood." [271] Let us study him now as he lays stress, not merely on the primacy of the blood, but on its psychological endowments.

Thirteen years before the date of Harvey's note-book Shakspere's play of "Hamlet" had appeared in print; in which the prince speaks thus of following his father's ghost: —

> "Why, what should be the fear?
> I do not set my life at a pin's fee;
> And, for my soul, what can it do to that,
> Being a thing immortal as itself?" [272]

It has been foreshadowed that for Harvey, the graduate of Cambridge and of Padua, the physician of the Renaissance, the word *"anima"* — "soul" — did not simply mean the immortal part of man, as for Hamlet, but was equivalent to the "*psyche*" of ancient philosophy. In order, therefore, readily to follow Harvey's thought at this juncture, we must first, like him, go to the fountain head; for only sayings of Aristotle can give us a sufficient clue to what he, and after him Harvey, meant by "soul."

Aristotle says in his treatise On Soul : —

"Some natural bodies have life and some have not. By life we mean the being nourished, and growing, and decaying, of oneself."

In the same treatise he says further : —

"The soul is that by which primarily we are alive, and display sensation and intellect; . . . but it is not matter and substratum."

Again he says : —

"Were the eye an animal, vision would be the soul thereof; for reason indicates that vision is the essence of the eye.[273] The eye in its turn is the material [basis] of vision; which latter failing, the eye is not an eye except in name, like an eye of stone or in a drawing."

The doctrines of the foregoing three passages are developed and made more explicit in the following, still from the treatise On Soul : —

"It is the presence of life, we say, which makes the difference between that which has soul and that which has not. To amplify regarding life: we call anything alive which possesses even a single one of the following: intellect, sensation, motion and rest in space, and also the motion [274] involved in nutrition, and both decay and growth. Therefore, even all the plants are held to be alive."

A few lines further on Aristotle says, speaking of the power or faculty [275] of taking nourishment : —

"This can exist without the others, but not the other faculties without this, in mortal beings. The aforesaid is clear in the case

of plants; for they possess no other faculty of the soul. To this
faculty then life owes its origin in living things; but the being an
animal owes its origin primarily to sensation; for beings that
neither move nor change their place but yet possess sensation, we
call animals and not merely living things. The primary sense,
which exists in all, is touch; and just as the nutritive faculty can
exist without touch or sensation of any kind, so can touch exist
without the other senses. The "nutritive" is our term for such
part of the soul as is shared even by plants, all animals, however,
evidently possessing the sense of touch. The cause of the presence
of each of the two aforesaid shall be told later. Now let us only
go so far as to say that the soul is the source of the [faculties] aforesaid, and is defined by means of them, to wit: the nutritive, the
sensory, the intellectual, the motor.[276] As to whether each of these
is a soul or is a part of the soul; and if a part, whether in the sense
that it is only separable by reasoning,[277] or locally as well — as to
some of these points, it is not hard to see our way, but some present
difficulties." [278]

If we turn to Aristotle's treatise On Generation we
find him dealing with the relations of the body to the
nutritive soul, in virtue whereof the body is alive;
with its relations to the sensory soul, in virtue whereof
it is an animal body; and, finally, in man with its relations to the intellectual soul. Of these three kinds of
soul or parts of the soul, he concludes, the mind "is
alone divine; for in the working thereof no bodily
working is involved." [279] Only soul of this divine
quality does he admit to be separable from body.[280]
The master has spoken. Now let the great pupil
speak. In the last Exercise but one of his treatise
On Generation, Harvey says, referring to the blood: —

"It assuredly contains the soul first and foremost, not only the
nutritive, but the sensory soul as well, and the motor. The blood
penetrates in all directions and is present everywhere; if it be

taken away, the soul itself is made away with also and at once; so
that the blood would seem to be wholly indistinguishable from the
soul or, at least, should be reckoned the substance of which the
soul is the activity.   The soul I aver to be such that neither is it
body at all, nor yet entirely without body, but comes in part from
without, in part is born on the premises,[281] and in a manner is part
of the body; in a manner, however, is the origin and cause of everything within the body of an animal, certainly of nutrition, sense,
and motion, and hence, in like manner, of life and death; for whatsoever is nourished, that same is living, and *vice versa*.   So, likewise, whatsoever is nourished abundantly, increases; but whatsoever too sparingly, dwindles; and whatsoever is nourished
perfectly, keeps its health; whatsoever otherwise, lapses into
disease.   Therefore, as is the soul, so also is the blood to be reckoned the cause and author of youth and old age, of sleep and of
waking, and even of respiration also — especially in view of this,
that in the things of nature the first instrument contains within
itself an internal moving cause.   Therefore, it comes to the same
whether one say that the soul and the blood, or the blood together
with the soul, or, if preferred, the soul together with the blood,
bring everything within an animal to pass." [282]

Only two years before these words were published the
aged Harvey had said the following: —

"Nor does the blood possess vigor, faculty, reason, motion, or
heat, as the gift of the heart." [283]

A comparison of the foregoing passages from Harvey
with the preceding passages from Aristotle makes it
clear that, for Harvey, although the soul dwells no
longer in its Aristotelian seat, it is no other than the
Aristotelian soul which pervades the "principal part"
of the body, the living blood of the Harveian circulation.

What proofs does Harvey offer that the soul is in the
blood? He has offered already one weighty piece of
evidence noted by many from of old in the chase, in

butchery, in sacrifice, in battle — the evidence from fatal hæmorrhage. This had been set forth nineteen centuries before him by one of his Hippocratic predecessors, who had referred to the reasoning

"used by those who say that the blood is the man ; for, seeing men slaughtered and the blood running out of the body, they conclude that the blood is the soul of man." [284]

Presently Harvey himself shall tell us that in placing the soul in the blood he is consciously reaffirming one of the most ancient of beliefs ; but he is far from basing his adhesion to it merely on such immemorial evidence, known to all, as the result of loss of blood, for he also adduces once more his own observations of the early embryo of the fowl, to prove not only the primacy of the blood but the presence of the soul therein. His testimony follows, and in reading it one must bear carefully in mind that in Harvey's time no clear scientific distinction had yet been worked out between movements which imply sensation, and movements, whether reflex or not, which do not depend upon consciousness. In his treatise On Generation Harvey says : —

"For my own part I am sure from numerous experiments that not only motion is inherent in the leaping point, — which no one denies — but sensation also. For you will see this point thrown into varied commotion and, as it were, irritated, at any touch whatever, even the slightest, just as sensitive bodies in general usually give evidence of sensation by movements proper to themselves. Moreover, if the injury be repeated often, the leaping point becomes excited and the rhythm and order of its pulsations disturbed. In like manner do we infer the presence of sensation in the so-called sensitive plant and in zoöphytes, from the fact that when they are

touched they draw themselves together as though taking it ill. . . .
So there is no doubt that the leaping point lives, moves, and feels
like an animal." [285]

In a later part of the same treatise he says : —

"It is manifest that all motion and sensation do not proceed from
the brain, since we plainly perceive the presence of motion and sensation before the brain has come into existence; what I have related proves that clearly sensation and motion dawn forthwith in
the first droplet of blood in the egg, before a vestige of the body
has been formed.   Moreover, in that first state of the structure or
constitution of the body which I have called the mucilaginous, before any members are discernible and when the brain is nothing but
limpid water, if the body be only lightly pricked it moves, contracts,
and twists itself obscurely like a worm or caterpillar; so that it
gives clear evidence of sensation." [286]

In another Exercise of the same treatise he says : —

"It is evident also from the generation of the chick, that whatever the source of its life or the vegetative first cause of it may
be, this had a prior existence in the heart.   Wherefore, if the said
first cause be itself the soul of the chick, it stands proved likewise
that this had a prior existence in the leaping point and the blood;
seeing that we observe therein motion and sensation; for it moves
and leaps like an animal.   If, then, there exist in the leaping point
the soul, which (as I have taught in my account) constructs for
itself the rest of the body, nourishes and increases it, certainly from
the heart as from a fount the soul flows out [287] into the entire body.

"So, likewise, if the egg be prolific because there is a soul in it,
or (as Aristotle would have it) the vegetative part of the soul, it is
clearly proved that the leaping point, in other words the generative
part endowed with soul, springs from the soul of the egg, for nothing
is the author of itself, and that the soul is transferred from the egg
to the leaping point, next to the heart, and then to the chick." [288]

In still another chapter of his treatise On Generation Harvey says : —

"Nor does the blood deserve to be called the original [289] part and the principal part, merely because in it and by it motion and pulsation are originated, but also because in the blood the psychical heat first comes into existence, the vital spirits are generated, and the soul itself inheres. For wherever the immediate and principal instrument of the vegetative faculty is first found, there probably the soul also is first present and takes its origin thence; since the soul is inseparable from the spirits and the innate heat. [290] . . .

"The life then inheres in the blood (as we read also in Holy Writ),[291] because therein the life and the soul are manifest first and fail last.[292] . . .

"It stands clearly proved that the blood is a generative part, the source of life, the first to live and the last to die, the primary seat of the soul; that in the blood, as in its source, the heat first and chiefly abounds and flourishes; and that by and from the blood all the other parts of the whole body are fostered and obtain their life by means of the influx of heat. Indeed, the heat which accompanies the blood floods, fosters, and preserves the entire body, as I have demonstrated already in my book on the motion of the blood." [293]

Harvey's proof that the blood is "the first to live and the last to die," we have scanned already in an earlier chapter of this paper. In the next chapter of his treatise On Generation he says : —

"No heat is to be found, either innate or inflowing, other than the blood, to be the soul's immediate instrument." [294]

On the next page, after briefly making certain suppositions, he says further : —

"Why should we not affirm with equal reason that there is soul in the blood; and also, since the blood is the first thing generated, nourished, and moved, that out of the blood the soul is first evoked and kindled? Certainly it is the blood in which vegetative and sensitive workings first come to light; in which heat, the primary and immediate instrument of the soul, is innate; it is the blood which is the common bond of body and soul, and in which as a vehicle soul flows into all parts of the whole body." [295]

But no matter how far on high the blood may have been exalted by Harvey the physician and psychologist, it is still subject to the lancet of Harvey the clinician, the heir of Hippocrates; for in his treatise On Generation, in the same Exercise with the foregoing passage, occurs the following : —

"While I assert that the seat of the soul is in the blood, first and foremost, I would not have the false conclusion drawn from this that all blood-letting is dangerous or hurtful; nor have it believed, as the multitude believes, that just to the degree that the blood is taken away does the life pass away at the same time, because holy scripture has placed the life in the blood. For it is known from everyday experience that the taking of blood is a wholesome aid against very many diseases and is chief among the universal remedies; seeing that depravity of the blood, or excess thereof, is at the bottom of a very great host of diseases; and that the timely evacuation of blood often brings exemption from most dangerous diseases and even from death itself. For just to the degree that the blood is taken away as our art prescribes, is an addition made to life and health. This very thing has been taught us by Nature, whom physicians set themselves to imitate; for Nature often makes away with the gravest affections by means of a large and critical evacuation by the nares, by menstruation, or by hæmorrhoids." [296]

Not only does Harvey affirm that "the soul is in the blood" and, as we have seen, appeal to observation and experiment in support of this doctrine; but he refers to those who had believed it before him, and maintains it against Aristotle's express denial. We have heard him testify as an observer; now let us hear him deal historically and polemically with the doctrine in question. Quite simply, in the final work of his old age, does the veteran tell of the wide acclaim which at last has greeted his discovery of the circulation — the most modern and revolutionary achievement of his time. The contrast is startling when, in the same breath, with equal simplicity he proceeds formally to identify his own latest view of the significance of the circulating blood with a doctrine which had been ancient in ancient times; a doctrine not only found in the Old Testament, but held by Greek thinkers who were historic figures even in the eyes of Aristotle. In his treatise On Generation Harvey says: —

"I see that the admirable circulation of the blood which I discovered long ago has proved satisfactory to nearly all, and that so far no one has made any objection to it which greatly calls for answer. Therefore, if I shall add the causes and uses of the circulation and reveal other secrets of the blood, showing how much it conduces to mortal happiness and to the welfare of soul as well as body, that the blood be kept pure and sweet by a right regimen, I truly believe that I shall do a work as useful and grateful to philosophers and physicians as it will be new; and that the following view will seem to nobody so improbable and absurd as it formerly seemed to Aristotle, viz.: that the blood, a domestic deity as it were, is the very soul within the body, as Critias and others thought of old; they 'believing that capacity for sensation is the most special attribute of the soul, and exists because of the nature of the blood.' By others again that which derives from its own nature the power of causing motion was held to be the soul; as Thales, Diogenes, Heraclitus, Alcmæon, and others believed.[297] It is made plain, however, by very numerous signs that both sensation and motion inhere in the blood in spite of Aristotle's [298] denial."[299]

We have noted with Harvey the doctrine of Leviticus, which still rules the procedure of the Jewish butcher;

and as we look backward to Athens across the centuries, we find Plato putting this question into the mouth of Socrates: "Whether it be the blood with which we think, or air, or fire, or none of these." [300] In Hellas this doctrine had been well known before Plato, Socrates, or the Hippocratic writers, one of whom we have found referring to it. The Sicilian Greek Empedocles, a philosopher and physician born at Acragas about 495 B.C., is said to have held, long before Aristotle, that the heart is the part formed first in the embryo; [301] and in a line of verse which has come down to us Empedocles said: "In the blood about man's heart is his understanding." [302] Empedocles is reported to have held to this because in the blood "are most perfectly blended the elements of the parts," [303] that is, earth, water, air, and fire.

The accomplished and wicked Athenian Critias, to whom Harvey refers, was that chief of the Thirty Tyrants who was slain in 403 B.C., four years before Socrates drank the hemlock and nineteen years before the birth of Aristotle. With the opinion of "Critias and others" Harvey, as we have seen, identifies his own view that the soul is in the blood. They held capacity for sensation to be the mark of soul and to be due to the nature of the blood; and Harvey's statement of these views is a literal quotation from the second chapter of the first book of Aristotle's treatise On Soul, which Harvey cites. This chapter is also the source of his summary and not quite exact reference to those other ancients who, as he avers, held spontaneous motor power to be the mark of soul — a power which Harvey unites in the blood with capacity for sensation. [304]

In the aforesaid chapter of Aristotle's work On Soul this philosopher had curtly reckoned among the "cruder" thinkers those of his predecessors who, "like Critias," had held the soul to be blood. Harvey notes the master's condemnation, but, as we have seen, stoutly ranges himself with the condemned ancients and affirms that sensation is inherent in the blood despite the master's denial. It is strange to note how the London physician seems less modern, for the moment, than the ancient philosopher of Athens. Aristotle, like a man of to-day, treats the blood simply as the immediate food of the tissues, noting expressly that it has "no feeling when touched in any animal, just as the excrement in the belly has no feeling." [305] Harvey deals as follows with this obvious truth in dealing with the question whether the blood can properly be reckoned a part of the body in the technical sense. He says : —

"At this time I will only say this : Even if we concede that the blood does not feel, nevertheless, it does not follow that it is not a part of a sensitive body and the principal part at that." [306]

We do not know that Aristotle ever saw or noted in the dying auricle the "undulation" by which Harvey was so much impressed ; but we have seen that, like Harvey, Aristotle treated of the development of the early embryo within the hen's egg and that, like Harvey, he laid special stress upon the red "leaping point." Aristotle concluded that the heart is the first generated living part, that it makes and will make throughout life the blood which it contains and distributes. In the heart he fixed the focus of the innate heat and, knowing nothing of the nervous system, he fixed in the heart the seat of the soul also. Harvey came to the conclusion that the blood is the first generated living part; that it has made the heart which contains it and which keeps it circulating and which it will nourish throughout life, as it will the other parts. In the blood itself he placed the innate heat and, though he knew the nervous system, he placed in the circulating blood the seat of the soul, which animates every part.

"We conclude," he says, "that the blood lives and is nourished of itself and in no wise depends upon any other bodily part either prior to or more excellent than itself." [307]

Thus the rigorously proved and demonstrated circulation of the blood was linked by its discoverer with the speculations of remote antiquity.

As we have seen, the use of the circulation became to Harvey a life-long subject of speculation, because this discovery had raised questions which no man could answer before the finding of oxygen. How obscure a problem Harvey found the functions of the blood to be, is nowhere better indicated than where he says in his old age : —

"So with better right one might maintain that the blood is equally the material of the body and its preserver, but not merely its food. For it is well known that in animals that perish of hunger, and also in men who waste away and die, there is abundance of blood to be found in the vessels, even after death." [308]

Is it the least part of Harvey's glory that his mind had cloven its way through long-lived beliefs to a truth which he could demonstrate but could not explain, and which seemed to other eminent men to be no truth, because too senseless to be true? [309]   When he finally broke with the ancient master, Harvey could not be content with sheer ignorance; and the same observations and experiments which led him out of Aristotelian error misled him into error quite as grave.   As to the venerable doctrine regarding the seat of the soul, which he at last embraced upon grounds now seen to be too slender, was not this doctrine one with which the Harveian circulation could harmonize well and which in turn could greatly glorify the circulation?   Let us pause, think, and read further.

CHAPTER X

THE BLOOD THE INNATE HEAT

THE latter part of Harvey's treatise On Generation is devoted to that of the mammal; but the treatise does not end with the end of this subject, for from his account of generation the author turns abruptly to append two Exercise on other topics. The first of these two is entitled "On the Innate Heat," and the second, which is very brief, is entitled "On the Primitive Moisture."

The Exercise On the Innate Heat is Harvey's express and polemical contribution to this subject, which had been much discussed both during and before his time;[310] a subject with which the famous discoverer deals roundly by maintaining that the innate heat is neither more nor less than the circulating blood. So the last words as to the significance of the circulating blood which he wrote for publication are contained in this Exercise. It begins as follows: —

"Since mention is often made of the innate heat, I propose now, by way of dessert, briefly to discuss the same and the primitive moisture also; and this the more willingly that I see there are many who take the greatest delight in those names and yet, in my judgment, comprehend but little of the things themselves. Truly, there is no need to seek for any spirits distinct from the blood, or to bring in heat from elsewhere, or call gods upon the stage and load philosophy with fanciful opinions; for what we so commonly would fetch from the stars is born at home. In truth, the blood alone is the innate warmth, or the first-born psychical heat; [311] as is proved excellently well by our observations of the generation of animals, especially of the chick in the egg; so that it were superfluous to multiply entities. Indeed, there is nothing to be met with in the animal body prior to the blood, or more excellent; nor are the spirits which they distinguish from the blood to be found anywhere separate from it; for the very blood itself, if without spirits or heat, does not deserve the name of blood, but of cruor. . . .

"Scaliger, Fernelius, and others lay less weight on the extraordinary endowments of the blood and imagine other spirits to exist, aërial or ethereal or composed of substance both ethereal and elemental, constituting an innate heat more excellent and more divine, as it were; and these spirits they believe to be the soul's most immediate instrument, the fittest for every use. They rely especially upon this argument, viz.: that the blood, being composed of elements, can exert no activity beyond the powers of the elements or of bodies consisting of a mixture thereof. Therefore, they imagine a spirit, another innate heat, of celestial origin and nature, to wit: a body most simple, most subtile, most fine, most mobile, most swift, most clear, ethereal, and sharing in the quintessence. Nowhere, however, has any such gift of spirit been demonstrated by them, nor that the same acts beyond the powers of the elements, or accomplishes greater works than could the blood alone. As for us who use our senses to guide us in the scrutiny of things, nowhere have we been able to find anything of the kind. Furthermore, there exist no cavities destined for the generation or preservation of these spirits, or even assigned thereto by the persons aforesaid." [312]

A little farther on we read : —

"I deem it, however, most wonderful that spirits which draw their origin from heaven and are adorned with such surpassing endowments should be nourished by our common and elemental air; especially seeing that their advocates hold that none of the elements can act beyond its own powers.[313] . . . What need then is there, say I, of that foreign guest, ethereal heat, since all can be accomplished by the blood, even as by it; while from the blood the spirits cannot withdraw a hair's breadth without perishing? Most assuredly nowhere do they wander or penetrate as separate bodies without the blood. For whether it be said that they are generated, nourished, and increased from the thinner part of the blood, as some believe, or from the primitive moisture, as others hold; yet it is confessed that they are never found outside the blood but forever cleave to the same as to their sustenance, as flame does to oil or to a wick. Wherefore their tenuity, subtility, mobility, and so forth, confer no greater advantage than does the blood which they continually accompany. It follows that the blood suffices and is fit to be the immediate instrument of the soul, since the blood is present everywhere and most swiftly permeates hither and thither." [314]

The two opponents named by Harvey were not his contemporaries, but worthies of the Renaissance who had written about one hundred years before the publication of his treatise On Generation and had died before he was born. The Italian physician Julius Cæsar Scaliger had written learned commentaries on Aristotle, as well as other works; and the Frenchman Jean Fernel, physician to King Henri II of France, had taught anatomy at Paris and had been a medical writer of importance. Each of these two authors was nearly sixty years of age in 1543, in which memorable year were first published the revolutionary writings of the aged astronomer Copernicus and of the young anatomist Vesalius, in the second year after the death of the hardy innovator Paracelsus. Such were the men against whose doctrines Harvey was impelled in his old age to launch his vigorous criticism, in order to clear the way for his own doctrine of the preëminence of the blood. What can we workers of to-day make of their opinions, which were living for Harvey but now are so deeply buried? Test-tube and balance, telescope, spectroscope, microscope, manometer, and the rest, have served their purpose so well since Harvey's time that even he, one of the foremost worthies of science, must seem merely to beat the air with words in his last message to us, unless we can recover his standpoint. Happily he himself shall attempt to clarify the meaning of his polemic by setting before us certain words of Aristotle, embodying far-reaching speculations as to body and soul in relation to the universe. Yet we shall find these not easy to understand.

Let Harvey continue his criticism of his predecessors. He says : —

"But while they believe that there are found in animals spirits and ultimate or primitive nourishment, or something else, which acts beyond the powers of the elements more than does the blood, they do not seem to have a sufficient grasp of what it may be to 'act beyond the powers of the elements'; nor have they rightly interpreted the words of Aristotle where he says: [315] 'The virtue or potency of every soul [316] seems to be associated with a body [317] other than the so-called elements and more divine.'"

And a little farther on : [318] —

"'For there exists in the semen of all [animals] that which makes their semen generative, the so-called heat. Yet this is not fire, nor any such power, but the spirits [319] included in the semen and in foaminess, and in the spirits the nature which is analogous to the element of the stars. [320] Wherefore fire generates no animal, nor does anything [animal] appear in process of formation in that, whether moist or dry, which is undergoing the action of fire; [321] whereas the heat of the sun and that of animals — not only that [which acts] through the semen, [322] but also, should there occur some excretion of a different nature [323] — even this, too, possesses a life-giving principle. It is patent, then, from such [facts] as these that the heat in animals is not fire and does not take its origin from fire.' [324]

"I, too, would say the same, for my part, of the innate heat and the blood, to wit: that it is not fire and does not take its origin from fire, but is associated with another body and that more divine, and, therefore, does not act by reason of any elemental faculty; but, just as there exists in the semen something which makes it generative and exceeds the powers of the elements in building an animal — to wit, spirits, and in the spirits a nature analogous [325] to the element of the stars — so likewise in the blood there exist spirits or some power which acts beyond the powers of the elements, a power very conspicuous in the nourishing and preserving of the several parts of an animal; and in the spirits and blood exist a nature, yea, a soul, analogous to the element of the stars. It is manifest, therefore, that the heat in the blood of animals during life is not fire and does not take its origin from fire; and this is taught excellently well by our own observations. [326] . . .

"Therefore, those who assert that nothing composed of the elements can work beyond the powers of these, unless it be associated at the same time with another body and that more divine, and maintain, therefore, that the spirits aforesaid consist in part of the elements, in part of some ethereal and celestial substance — truly, such persons seem to me to have drawn their conclusions ill. For you shall find scarcely any elemental body which, when in action, will not exceed its own proper powers." [327]

On reaching the end of the last quoted words of Harvey's polemic, a physician or biologist of to-day may easily be conscious of disappointment, even of a mild despair; for the once celebrated passage from Aristotle, about the interpretation of which Harvey gives battle, seems at first the source of all the obscurities of the controversy, rather than of the promised light which shall clear them away. Yet that light must come by way of that rugged passage. The gist of the first part of the Aristotelian passage may be set forth as follows: In the semen soul is potential, being associated therein with a "body" or "nature" which possesses a "life-giving principle" and is in the spirits, *i.e.*, in the hot vapor, within the foam-bubbles of the semen. This body or nature is called heat, yet it is not that one of the four elemental bodies which is known as fire, nor yet a derivative of this, but is "a body other than the so-called elements and more divine," a "nature analogous to the element of the stars." What is this "element of the stars"? It is clear that only from the answer to this question can the light which we are seeking begin to shine. To find this celestial element we must immediately take a rapid glance at the Aristotelian universe — that grand conception which the master mainly accepted from his predecessors and contemporaries, but owed, in part, to the work of his own mind. Let us swiftly scan what he styled the "Cosmos."

At the center thereof is the earth, spherical and motionless. The core of the universe consists not only of this central globe with everything in or upon it, but also of the atmosphere or, more correctly, of all which extends between the surface of the globe and the nearest of the distant revolving hollow spheres of heaven, in some of which spheres are set the heavenly bodies. Below the heavenly spheres this core of the universe is made up of the four elements, earth, water, air, and fire; and all things composed of these are subject to opposed and limited and compounded motions, to generation, alteration, and corruption. The inclosing heaven, on the other hand, is unchangeable and eternal, has never been created, and will never be destroyed. Its many component hollow spheres are contiguous and concentric, and concentric also with our globe. In a single sphere, the outermost, called the "first heaven,"

all the fixed stars are set.   In separate spheres, nearer
to the earth, are set the seven bodies which the astronomy of Aristotle's day styled "planets."   To
these (here designated by their present names) that
ancient astronomy assigned the following order from
the earth outward toward the fixed stars : the moon, the
sun, Venus, Mercury, Mars, Jupiter, and Saturn.
Each of the celestial spheres revolves with simple circular motion in one direction forever.   The "first
heaven," the sphere of the fixed stars, needs but the
one simple motion which is its own, and it carries with
it in its daily revolution all the inner spheres.   These
are more numerous than the seven planets ; for though
each planet is set in but a single sphere, each planet's
complex course results from the combined simple motions of more spheres than one.   In spite of these
more or less intimate relations, the spheres of heaven
are separate existences, self-moved, like animals ; and,
like animals, possess activity, life, and soul.   But the
motion and life of the heavenly existences are continuous and eternal, and hence these existences — the
spheres, and the planets and fixed stars set therein —
are all divine ; much more divine than man, though
man possesses a far larger share of the divine than
other animals.[328]

Just as the troubled regions which lie below the
sphere of the moon are contrasted with the serene
heaven which incloses and limits them, so the changing
forms of matter which compose our globe and its nearer
surroundings are contrasted with the simple unalterable
substance of the heavenly spheres.   "Of necessity,"
says Aristotle, "there exists a simple body whose very

nature it is to be borne on in circular motion." [329]
Elsewhere he says that the men of old "would seem to
have assumed that the body which moves forever is
likewise divine by nature." [330]   This is "an embodied
substance different from the compounds here, more
divine and prior to them all"; [331] a body "of a nature
the more precious the farther it is withdrawn from what
is here." [332]   After reasoning about this body Aristotle
says : —

"If what has been laid down be accepted, it is plain from the
foregoing why the first of bodies is eternal, and shows neither
growth nor decay nor old age nor alteration, and is affected by
nothing.   The conception seems to testify to the phenomena and the
phenomena to the conception. . . .   Therefore, as the first body
is something different from earth and fire and air and water, [the
ancients] gave the name of ether to the region most on high, naming
it from its moving always during all eternity." [333]

The place in nature of "the first element," so grandly
conceived, is fixed more definitely by Aristotle when he
says "that the whole universe in the region of the
courses on high is filled with that body." [334]

Now, therefore, we have attained the object of our
rapid quest ; at last we have reached "the element of
the stars"; for Aristotle tells us that not only heaven,
but all the heavenly bodies as well, consist of the
ether, saying : —

"It is most reasonable and consequent, in view of things already
said, for us to make each of the stars out of that body in which it
has its course, since we have declared the existence of something
of which the nature is to be borne in a circle." [335]

At a later day the ethereal element of the stars was distinguished from the four inferior elements not by its

Aristotelian name of first element but by that of fifth element, or fifth existence, or fifth "essence." Hence arose and was applied to the fifth element the name "quintessence"; a word which in its turn acquired various meanings.

Ten years after Harvey's death Milton published his description of the creation of heaven; a description couched, however, in terms of the uncreated heaven of Aristotle.   Milton wrote: —

> "And this ethereal quintessence of heaven
> Flew upward, spirited with various forms,
> That roll'd orbicular, and turned to stars
> Numberless, as thou seest, and how they move;
> Each had his place appointed, each his course;
> The rest in circuit walls this universe." [336]

We may now return from this excursion through the "Cosmos," to bring its light to bear upon those high-sounding words of Aristotle which, according to Harvey, formed the basis of speculations about the innate heat, the spirits, and the blood, which were handed down by "Scaliger, Fernelius, and others," and affected the views of Harvey himself.   Aristotle had written: —

> "The virtue or potency of every soul [316] seems to be associated with a body [317] other than the so-called elements, and more divine."

And a little farther on: —

> "For there exists in the semen of all [animals] that which makes their semen generative, the so-called heat.   Yet this is not fire, nor any such power, but the spirits [319] included in the semen and in foaminess, and in the spirits the nature which is analogous to the element of the stars." [337]

That generative heat which is not elemental fire, but a "body" or "nature" diviner than the lower elements, can be the analogue of nothing else than the celestial ether.

What led Aristotle to so lofty a flight of speculation? He does not tell. One may guess, however, that it may well have been this: that he had found himself obliged not only to deny the identity of the generative heat of the semen with elemental fire, but also to deny the identity with elemental fire even of the glowing sun, as well as of the other planets and the fixed stars; and to maintain that all the heavenly bodies consist of ether. These denials we have read already; they shall presently be commented on. Taking them for granted: now, since the life-giving sun is not elemental fire but ether, would not the life-giving seminal heat, which also is not elemental fire, naturally be the analogue of the ether? "Man and the sun generate man," said Aristotle, in a famous passage.[338] He needed no knowledge of chlorophyll to teach him this. The ether is the element of the sun, moon, stars, and spheres; of it consist the bodies associated with the souls of the living, unalterable, immortal, divine existences of the eternal heaven. To associate a body analogous to this ether with the dormant soul of a living existence — a living existence alterable and mortal as an individual, but one of an immortal race — in the medium which shall maintain that racial immortality by begetting a new individual out of the lower elements — this is a stroke characteristic of the man who declared that "the race of men, and of animals, and of plants, exists forever"; [339] the man who assigned to every bloodless animal an analogue of the blood and an analogue of the heart,[340] to the octopus, an analogue of the brain; [341] the man in whose eyes the heavenly bodies were divine living existences running eternal courses and so, we may presume, were analogous in some degree to the living existences of the earth.[342]

Harvey in one of the earlier Exercises of his treatise On Generation had already followed the ancient master's footsteps in this matter. Discoursing of the endless succession of generations the pupil says that this

"makes the race of fowls eternal; since now the chick and now the egg, in an ever-continued series, produce an immortal species out of individuals which fail and perish. We discern, too, that in similar fashion many lower things rival the perpetuity of higher things. And whether or no we say that there is a soul in the egg, it clearly appears from the cycle aforesaid that there underlies this revolution from hen to egg and from egg again to hen, a principle which bestows eternity upon them. That same, according to Aristotle,[343] is analogous to the element of the stars; and it makes parents generate, makes their semen or eggs prolific, and, like Proteus, is ever present."[344]

Let us return now to Harvey's polemic. In it he does not give chapter and verse by which we can properly verify more than a few of his statements of the views of "Scaliger, Fernelius, and others"; but the words of Aristotle which Harvey quotes go far to justify his intimation that the views which he states and combats, as the champion of the circulating blood, are largely derived from those Aristotelian words — whether by misinterpretation, as he roundly but indefinitely declares, or with deliberate modification of doctrine, need not now concern us.

At the very outset of Harvey's discourse about the innate heat, the first doctrine that he reprobates is a striking one, viz.: that the innate heat is one and the same thing with spirits distinguishable from the blood, though not separable from it. Of these spirits he stoutly denies the existence, on the true scientific ground of lack of all evidence from observation in their favor. Our earlier studies of ancient doctrines of respiration have brought before us, as supposed to exist in the blood, spirits variously styled "elemental," "aërial," "nourished by our common and elemental air," "nourished and increased from the thinner part of the blood." We have even read Galen's words of spirits which are "the soul's most immediate instrument," viz.: the "animal spirits" in the brain and nerves. Indeed, during the eighteen centuries between the death of Aristotle and the boyhood of Fernelius and Scaliger, the word "*pneuma*" — "spirits" or "spirit" — did most varied duties in the service of physicians, philosophers, alchemists, and theologians; and this same word is of great importance in the scriptures.[345] It is noticeable that, although Harvey rejects the doctrine of spirits in the blood, even he himself talks of the blood being itself spirits.[346] This fact, however, should not militate against him or lead to confusion. The word "spirits" being a very comprehensive technical term of his day, he does not refuse to employ it as a label for qualities of the blood after he has denied the very existence of what is properly denoted by the word "spirits." He simply behaves as we behave when we talk of the "sympathetic" nerves, though the theory is exploded which the adjective expresses; or when we speak of "animal cell," well knowing that no proper wall necessarily surrounds the living substance.

Despite the protean forms of the spirits it is not till

we have reached Harvey's Exercise On the Innate Heat
that we have fallen in with spirits in the blood which, for
some of his predecessors, "constitute an innate heat
more excellent and more divine, as it were"; nor with
"a spirit, another innate heat, of celestial origin and
nature." For this treatment of spirits within the blood
and of innate heat, as convertible terms, the way may
well have been paved by the words in which Aristotle
intimates that the generative heat of the semen resides
in the spirits therein, i.e., in hot vapor produced within
the body of the male and included within the films of
foam-bubbles in the semen. Referring to "the so-
called heat" the words of Aristotle are: "Yet this is
not fire nor any such power, but the spirits included in
the semen and in foaminess, and in the spirits the
nature which is analogous to the element of the stars."[347]
The transition can hardly have been too difficult from
the view of Aristotle that in the spirits of the semen is
heat which is not elemental fire, to the view combated
by Harvey that the spirits of the blood are heat which is
not elemental fire.

Aristotle's striking biological doctrine that the generative seminal heat is a "nature which is analogous to
the element of the stars" appears to be an obvious
source of those seeming fantasies, written down eighteen
centuries later, at which Harvey girds when he says:
"For what we so commonly would fetch from the stars
is born at home." If we use our judgment simply,
upon Harvey's statement of their opinions, the men
whom he castigates, having strayed from the ancient
master's footsteps by making the spirits one and the
same with the innate heat instead of the vehicle thereof,

next stray still more blindly by identifying this heat, *alias* these spirits, not with an analogue of the ether, but with a portion of the ether itself. Therefore is it that we read in the words of Harvey's polemic, of "that foreign guest, ethereal heat"; of those spirits "aërial or ethereal, or composed of substance both ethereal and elemental"; of spirits "which draw their origin from heaven" and elicit Harvey's ironical wonder that they "should be nourished by our common and elemental air." Therefore, too, is he able to tell us of that amazing spirit, *alias* innate heat, which is "a body" and qualified by many imposing adjectives and finally styled "ethereal and sharing in the quintessence." The doctrine of Aristotle that in the semen there are spirits which are the vehicle of generative heat which is analogous to the element of the stars, is a baseless doctrine, but it is a subtle and far-reaching speculation. The doctrine stated and attacked by Harvey that in the blood there are spirits which are the innate heat, which consists as a whole or in part of the element of the stars, is not only a baseless doctrine, as Harvey vigorously shows, but certainly is lame as speculation despite its glittering appeal to the imagination. To make spirits and innate heat convertible terms may pass as but one among many phases of speculation. But to bring down actual ether from heaven to earth, although attempted by eminent thinkers [348] centuries before Scaliger and Fernelius, is to bring chaos into that conception of the universe which requires the "first element" to revolve forever on high, above that lower world which lies beneath the sphere of the moon. To Aristotle such chaos surely would have been abhorrent; indeed, it runs counter to his expressed description of the ether.[349] Moreover, Aristotle's application of the term "analogue" to the generative heat is equivalent to a denial that the generative heat is actually ether; for analogues do frequent service in his doctrines and he explicitly states the analogue of a thing to be something different from the thing itself.[350] What that mysterious analogue of the ether may be with which the generative heat is identified we are not explicitly told, as we are not told what the analogue of the heat may be in bloodless animals.   We are left to judge for ourselves after deeper investigation of nature or deeper study of the Aristotelian writings.   Had Aristotle been ready to define and describe the body which is more divine than the four lower elements, but is not the first element on high, he probably would not have chosen an analogue as the fittest vehicle for his thought.

According to Harvey the horse of battle of his criticized predecessors was the argument stated by him as follows: "That nothing composed of the elements can work beyond the powers of these, unless it be associated at the same time with another body and that more divine; and . . . therefore, that the spirits aforesaid consist in part of the elements, in part of some ethereal and celestial substance." [351]   The "spirits aforesaid" are held to be one and the same with the innate heat and reside in the blood.   Aristotle had written, we remember: "The virtue or potency of every soul seems to be associated with a body other than the so-called elements and more divine," [352] viz.: the generative seminal heat, which is not fire but an analogue of the ether.   It would seem fairly probable that largely from this doctrine of Aristotle was developed the doctrine about the "powers of the elements" which Harvey sets forth in his polemic. Nothing can be more emphatic than his disagreement with the advocates of this doctrine. "Such persons," he says, "seem to me to have drawn their conclusions ill. For you shall find scarcely any elemental body which, when in action, will not exceed its own proper powers." [353] On the same page with this sweeping statement we find it supported by the following very simple line of thought : —

"All natural bodies present themselves in a double relation, to wit : according as they are reckoned with apart and comprehended within the circuit of their own proper nature, or according as they are the instruments of some nobler and superior authority. For, as to their own proper powers, there is no doubt that all things which are subject to generation and corruption derive their origin from the elements, and work according to the standard thereof. In so far, however, as all things so subject are instruments of a more excellent agent and are regulated thereby, their works do not proceed from their own proper nature but from the rule of that other ; and, consequently, they seem to be associated with another and more divine body and to exceed the powers of the elements." [354]

In the very next Exercise, however, that On the Primitive Moisture, the last Exercise of Harvey's treatise On Generation, we come suddenly upon a reason why "the powers of the elements" must have seemed to him something to be treated rather as a convenient form of words than as a serious doctrine, despite his respectful argument just quoted. Speaking of the "primitive moisture," the great observer says that he sees in the hen's egg that out of that "crystalline colliquament," that "simplest body" alone, all the parts of the embryo are made and increased; [355] and proceeds bluntly to question the reality of the elements, "namely, the fire, air, water, and earth of Empedocles and Aristotle; or the salt, sulphur, and mercury of the chemists; or the atoms of Democritus." [356]   Harvey says : —

"Therefore, the so-called elements do not exist prior to whatever is generated or arises; but rather are subsequent thereto, being remains rather than origins. Not even Aristotle himself, nor any one else, has ever demonstrated that elements exist separately in nature, or give rise to bodies which consist of parts similar one to another." [357]

Almost immediately after this tug at the foundations of the Aristotelian universe, Harvey brings his treatise On Generation to an end.

The admirable feature of Harvey's brief last-published discussion of the circulating blood is this, that the aged veteran ever strikes vigorous blows for observation, for the use of the senses, in the search for truth. But we have seen already that by his arm, as by another's, the blows are delivered both for better and for worse.   Rightly does he drive out of court the spirits "ethereal and elemental" which no man can demonstrate.   Wrongly does he discredit the real complexity of that humor, to the eye so simple and crystal-clear, out of which he believes all the diverse parts of the living bird to be developed.   In Harvey's present polemic we find no new appeal to nature; he vindicates the justice of his former appeals and maintains with vigor the doctrines already familiar to us, that the blood is the principal part of the body, is itself the innate heat, and is the seat of the soul.   This relation of blood and soul he reaffirms very impressively in this, his final public utterance; a most important passage of which, about the presence of the soul in the blood, has been embodied in the chapter on that subject of the present paper.[358]

But evidently the main purpose of his polemical Exercise on the Innate Heat is to cast out of the blood the futile spirits which obscure the real relation of that heat to the circulating blood; and so to defend the thesis best set forth in the following words of his own : —

"In truth, the blood alone is the innate warmth, or the first born psychical heat; as is proved excellently well by our observations of the generation of animals, especially of the chick in the egg; so that it were superfluous to multiply entities.[359] . . . What need, then, is there, say I, of that foreign guest, ethereal heat, since all can be accomplished by the blood, even as by it?"[360]

Harvey has expelled from the blood the mythical spirits which had stood in the way of the direct identification of the blood with the innate heat. But how does he interpret the famous words of Aristotle which he quotes, and declares not to have been "rightly interpreted" by the champions of ethereal spirits? When we seek an answer to this question, we do not find the veteran discoverer at his best. The ancient philosopher surely would have been as much surprised at Harvey's interpretation of his words as at any use of them made by Scaliger or Fernelius. We have seen that Harvey follows up his quotation from Aristotle by promptly applying its language, literally or by paraphrase, to the innate heat and the blood.[361] Emphatic

are the words which immediately follow the words of
Aristotle.   Harvey says : —

"I, too, would say the same, for my part, of the innate heat and
the blood, to wit : that it is not fire and does not take its origin
from fire, but is associated with another body and that more
divine."

This denial he soon repeats, adding the words : "and
this is taught excellently well by our observations."

According to Aristotle the soul in the semen is associated with a body diviner than the four lower elements,
viz. : the generative heat, an analogue of the element
of the stars, which analogue resides in spirits, *i.e.*, in
hot vapor within bubbles of seminal foam.   In the case
of the blood, according to Harvey, it is the heat itself,
the innate heat *alias* the blood, which is associated
with "another body and that more divine," and Harvey,
having denied the reality of the spirits, uses the word
"spirits" as equivalent to "some power" in the blood,
which power is "very conspicuous in the nourishing and
preserving of the several parts of an animal."   In the
spirits, so understood, and the blood, dwells the soul ;
and it is the soul itself which Harvey states to be "a
nature analogous [*respondens* not *proportione respondens*] to the element of the stars."   Even as the word
"spirits" has become, in effect, a label for powers of
the blood, so the analogue of the ether becomes, in
effect, a pious epithet applied to the soul ; and only to
the soul itself can Harvey have referred as "another
body and that more divine."   In the next page to the
passage now under discussion he says : —

"The blood, therefore, is spirits, because of its extraordinary virtues and powers. It is also celestial, inasmuch as in the spirits aforesaid is lodged a nature, the soul, to wit, which is analogous to the element of the stars; something, that is, analogous to heaven, the instrument of heaven, vicarious of heaven.[362] . . . The heat of the blood is psychical, inasmuch as it is governed in its operations by the soul;[363] it is also celestial, because subservient to heaven; and divine, because the instrument of God, the best and greatest.[364] . . . The lower world, according to Aristotle, is so connected with the courses on high that all its motives and changes seem to take thence their origin and to be governed thence.[365] Truly, in that world which the Greeks called the 'Cosmos' from the beauty of its order,[366] lower and corruptible things are subject to other higher and incorruptible things; but all are beneath the highest, the omnipotent and eternal Creator, and obey Him."[367]

It is obvious that, although Harvey in dealing with the blood does not forego the use of the phrases used by the ancient master in dealing with the semen, nevertheless, the entities recognized by Harvey are not only fewer than those of Aristotle, but are differently disposed within the draperies of Aristotelian language. Harvey's entities are simply the innate heat *alias* the blood, and the soul which dwells therein; but he sincerely takes himself to be an interpreter of Aristotle's words, as appears a second time from an echo of those words which we meet in an earlier Exercise of Harvey's treatise On Generation. Here, pleading that it is true that the soul is in the blood, Harvey refers to Aristotle by name and immediately says : —

"Indeed, if he is constrained by the truth to acknowledge that there is a soul in an egg, even in a wind-egg;[368] and that in the semen and the blood also there is found something which is divine and analogous to the element of the stars and is vicarious of the omnipotent Creator; and if certain of the moderns truly say," etc., etc.[369]

These zealous words show Harvey drawn into statements by no means warranted by the text of Aristotle. We have seen that the Aristotelian heaven was uncreated;[370] and, whatever Harvey in his day may have thought, no "omnipotent Creator" is revealed by more modern study of the Aristotelian philosophy. Whatever inferences Harvey may have drawn from Aristotle's words, Aristotle does not "acknowledge"[371] that the analogue of the ether exists in the blood. Moreover, when in Harvey's Exercise On the Innate Heat that analogue of the element of the stars which Aristotle associated with the soul is identified by Harvey with the soul itself, the change is almost as great as if one should declare that protoplasm is life, instead of styling it with Huxley "the physical basis of life." In a third Exercise of the treatise On Generation, the earliest of the three, Harvey had dealt in a better and more characteristic way with the analogue of the ether; though here, too, his exposition gives no accurate idea of Aristotle's doctrine. In discussing Aristotle's opinion as to how the semen of the cock causes the formation of the embryo Harvey says of Aristotle: —

"Indeed, where he appears to settle and determine with certainty what that may be in whatsoever seed, whether of plants or of animals, which renders the same fruitful, he rejects heat and fire as unfit for the work, but does not give recognition to any similar faculty, nor yet discover in the seed aught suitable for that duty; but is forced to admit something incorporeal, and coming from without, which shall act with understanding and foresight (like art or mind) to form the foetus, and therein shall establish and order all things to a purpose and for the better. He betakes himself, I say, to something obscure and to us unknown, 'spirits included in the semen and in foaminess, and in the spirits the nature which is analogous to the element of the stars.' But what that may be he has nowhere taught us." [372]

We have found that Aristotle describes "the element of the stars" as a "body," [373] and that in the passage about the semen which Harvey quotes Aristotle expressly applies the same term, "body," to the analogue of the element of the stars. [374] Yet to this analogue Harvey seems to refer as "something incorporeal" in his last-quoted words, which tend to confound it with soul. Harvey agrees with Aristotle, however, in calling fire a "body"; [375] and where in his Exercise On the Innate Heat he extols at some length [376] fire, air and water in motion as flame, wind and flood, he also sets forth how they each claim the title of spirits "by virtue of their movement and perpetual flux," [377] and says : —

"These three, therefore, in so far as they acquire a certain life, appear to act beyond the powers of the elements and to have a share [378] of another and diviner body; wherefore they were reckoned among the deities by the heathen. For that of which the outcome is some extraordinary work, exceeding the bare faculties of the elements, that same they held to proceed from some diviner agent; as though it were one and the same to act beyond the powers of the elements and to have a share of another and diviner body — diviner, because it does not derive its origin from the elements." [379]

Nowhere but in the third chapter of the second book of Aristotle's treatise On Generation does he refer to the analogue of the ether ; and the complete text of this chapter — rugged, here and there, especially in Gaza's Latin translation — may help us perhaps to account for some of Harvey's efforts at exposition.[380]   But when these and his reports of his predecessor's doctrines are compared with the words of Aristotle, Harvey and those other biologists of the Renaissance seem like sturdy children reaching forward in the dust, each still clasping a finger of the strong old father who strides among them.

CHAPTER XI

So Harvey denies the doctrine falsely based upon
Aristotle's words, the doctrine of the ethereal nature
of the innate heat; but he affirms and adopts as his
own the Aristotelian distinction between the heat which
is sterile and the heat which gives life. This weighty
affirmation obliges us who study Harvey to examine
this impressive distinction further.[381]

Aristotle says, we remember: "The heat in animals
is not fire and does not take its origin from fire." We
remember also that Harvey says: "I, too, would say
the same, for my part, of the innate heat and the blood,
to wit: that it is not fire and does not take its origin
from fire." This doctrine is based by both Aristotle
and Harvey upon observation; and Aristotle's argument is contained in the passage which Harvey quotes,
a passage obscure in the Latin and rugged in the Greek.
Briefly, Aristotle's argument is this: Observation shows
that fire is sterile, but that the heat of the sun is generative and the heat of animals likewise; therefore, the heat
of animals is not fire. Harvey declares that this same
conclusion "is taught excellently well" by his observations also — by which he does not expressly say. That
Aristotle, in drawing the distinction aforesaid between
the heat of fire and the heat of the sun, was playing at

hide and seek with a great truth of biology, would soon be apparent to whosoever should take a flourishing green plant from a window warmed by sunshine and try to make the same plant flourish in a dark room warmed by a hidden fire.

At this point let us scan further the words of Aristotle which Harvey has quoted.[337]   Aristotle says : [318] —

"For there exists in the semen of all [animals] that which makes their semen generative, the so-called heat. Yet this is not fire, nor any such power, but the spirits [319] included in the semen and in foaminess, and in the spirits the nature which is analogous to the element of the stars.[320] Wherefore fire generates no animal, nor does anything [animal] appear in process of formation in that, whether moist or dry, which is undergoing the action of fire ; [321] whereas the heat of the sun and that of animals — not only that [which acts] through the semen, [322] but also, should there occur some excretion of a different nature [323] — even this, too, possesses a life-giving principle. It is patent, then, from such [facts] as these that the heat in animals is not fire and does not take its origin from fire." [324]

In this passage a forcible presentment is made of the sterilizing power of fire, and elsewhere we are told by Aristotle that "only in earth and in water are there animals ; there are none in air and in fire." [382] That by the word "fire" we are to understand elemental heat of greater or less intensity is sufficiently shown perhaps by the context. But no doubt will linger if we glance at two lines from another treatise in which, referring expressly to the four elements, Aristotle speaks of earth, water, air, and "what as a matter of custom we call 'fire,' but it is not fire ; for fire is an excess, a boiling, as it were, of heat." [383]

Harvey, looking askance as he did at the four ancient elements and even bluntly questioning the elementary

constitution of matter, felt himself free to reduce the
analogue of the ether to a pious epithet, and yet to
accept with emphasis the Aristotelian doctrine that the
heat of animals "is not fire."   At the end of his Exercise On the Primitive Moisture he says: "Nor, lastly,
do we find that anything is naturally generated out of
fire, as out of something capable of mixture, and the
thing is perhaps impossible."   Here, however, he is not
dealing merely with the generation of living beings, but
with a subject deeper yet, the possibility of fire acting
as an element at all.[384]

The drift of those sentences which Harvey quotes is
lighted up, better perhaps than by any modern commentary, by a passage of Cicero's treatise On the Nature of the Gods, a treatise mentioned by Harvey in
his lecture notes,[385] as we have seen.   In the orator's
lucid Latin we may read what purports to be a quotation
from the Greek philosopher Cleanthes, who was a child
when Aristotle died in 322 B.C., and who became the
second head of the Stoic school, the powerful younger
rival of the school of Aristotle.   Let us listen to the
Roman stoic of 45 or 44 B.C., who is set up by Cicero
to quote and expound Cleanthes as follows: —

"Cleanthes says: 'Since the sun is fiery and is nourished by
the humors of Ocean (seeing that no fire can last without some kind
of food), therefore, the sun must needs be similar either to the fire
which we use and apply in our daily life, or to that fire which is
contained in the bodies of animate beings.   But this fire of ours,
which is requisite for the uses of life, is the destroyer and consumer
of all things, and wheresoever it has made its way disturbs and
dissipates everything; whereas that fire of the body is vital and
salutary and by it everything is preserved, nourished, increased,
sustained, and endowed with sense.'   Cleanthes denies, therefore,

that it is doubtful to which of these two fires the sun is similar, seeing that the sun likewise makes all things flourish and ripen, each after its kind. Wherefore, since the sun's fire is similar to those fires which exist in the bodies of animate beings, the sun, too, must be an animate being and, indeed, the rest of the stars that arise in the celestial ardor which is named ether or heaven." [386]

Unlike Aristotle, Cicero's stoic admits that the sun and even the heavenly ether are fire. But we see him to be no less impressed than Aristotle by the difference between the killing heat of flame and the life-giving heat of heaven and of living things. It is interesting to find this difference expressly given as a reason for believing the heavenly bodies to be alive; and one wonders whether this difference may not have had some share in convincing Aristotle that the ether is an element distinct from fire and the other three elements, and more exalted than they. It must be said. however, that Aristotle's habitual use of language about "the heat contained in animals" prepares us ill for the momentous distinction drawn by him between this and elemental heat.

We have found him speaking of "the soul being, as it were, afire" within the heart; [387] and he says also that "the concoction through which nutrition takes place in animals does not go on either in the absence of soul or in the absence of heat, seeing that everything is done by fire." [388]   Moreover, there is in his treatise On Soul a passage deserving immediate quotation, no less as a picture of the nascent stage of biological thought, than as showing a phase of Aristotelian doctrine contrasting with the doctrine of the analogue of the ether. He says : —

"By some the nature of fire is held to be quite simply the cause of nutrition and growth; for fire alone among bodies or elements is seen being nourished and growing; wherefore one might assume it to be that which does the work both in plants and in animals. It is, in a way, the contributing cause [389] but not the cause in the simple sense, the soul rather being that; for the growth of fire is limitless, so long as there are combustibles, but in the case of all natural organisms [390] there is a limit to size and growth, and a rationale [391] thereof; these things depending upon the soul, not upon fire, and upon reason rather than upon matter." [392]

Nevertheless, in spite of seeming inconsistencies, we find Aristotle declaring that the heat of fire sterilizes, but the heat of the sun and of animals gives life. Moreover, when he tells us in the passage quoted by Harvey [393] that not only the heat of the sun and of semen, but also the heat of other animal excretions possesses a "life-giving principle," the words appear to suggest not merely generation without sex, but the spontaneous generation either of parasites within the animal body, or of living things in matters cast off from it. We seem to be confronted with the far-reaching thought that there is in the world a life-giving principle by which, when associated with soul, matter is quickened in ways of which sexual generation is only one; and that this principle is generative heat, streaming from the sun or transmitted by the male in coition, and, thereafter, innate in the resulting creature and shared by the humors thereof. The fact must always have been recognized that in some way the existence of living things on earth depends upon the sun. On the other hand, no modern methods fortified Aristotle's intelligence against spontaneous generation, which he accepted as a matter of course and called "automatic generation," even asserting that eels and some other fishes originate in this way.[394]   Further statements of his own shall show us now that the sun in its orbit dominates the changes upon and above the earth and is the giver of life, whether imparted by sexual intercourse or otherwise.   Then Harvey shall repeat the lesson and thus help us to understand his declaration regarding the innate heat and the blood, to wit: that it "is not fire and does not take its origin from fire."

Aristotle refers to a region beneath the celestial spheres, which region he calls "the first in proximity to the earth," or "the region common to water and air." He says of the events therein : —

"Of these the efficient [395] cause and ruler and first origin is the circle of the sun's course, which, it is evident, produces separation and combination by its approach or withdrawal and is the cause of generation and corruption." [396]

These last words are used in a large sense to mean the formation and disintegration of whatever is composed of the four elements.

But the annual circuit of the sun does more than bring to pass the rhythmic changes of the seasons with their effects upon man's environment.   To the sun's circuit man owes his life.   Aristotle has said to us already: "Man and the sun generate man," in words which have no biological context.[338]   He does better when he enumerates among the "causes" of a man these three: his father, the sun, and "the oblique circle," *i.e.*, the ecliptic.   These he styles "efficient [397] causes" of man, [398] as we have heard him style "the circle of the sun's course" the "efficient cause" of the mighty changes in inanimate things.   We learn in

what sense a father is the "efficient cause" of his off-
spring when Aristotle says: "The female always
provides the matter, while the male provides that which
fashions it"; [399] and when we are told that this matter
provided by the female "is quickened by the principle
derived from the male, which thus perfects the
animal"; [400] "the animal" meaning the product of
conception. "The body," says Aristotle further, "is
from the female, but the soul from the male." [401]   For
although he says elsewhere that "Genesis is the first
obtaining in heat of a share of nutritive soul, and life
is the tarrying thereof"; [402] although he concedes a
share of this lowest kind of soul to wind-eggs, to plants,
and to the humblest things which live; nevertheless,
he holds that, where the sexes are divided, the indispensable "sensory soul" which distinguishes the animal
from the plant is derived from the male parent only.[403]
So the seminal fluid and the solar rays are coupled together as "efficient causes" of man; and thus the
moving sun is made responsible, by what chain of
causation we are not told expressly, for the results of
sexual generation.

From this we may turn now to other forms of generation in the light of the following prodigious analogy.
Aristotle says: —

"We call 'male' an animal which engenders within another,
and 'female' one which engenders within itself; and, therefore,
in the case of the universe the earth's nature is held to be female
and maternal, while heaven and the sun and other such are called
engenderers and fathers." [404]

Next, after these sweeping generalities, let us peruse Aristotle's account of spontaneous generation.   He says: —

"Animals and plants arise in earth and in moisture, because in earth there is water and in water there is air,[319] and in all air there is psychical heat; so that in a certain sense all things are full of soul. Therefore, when once inclusion of this [405] has taken place, an individual is quickly formed.[406] Inclusion takes place and a kind of foam-bubble arises, produced by the heating of moisture which has body [407] of its own." [408]

The last expression in this passage evidently means moisture which is charged with earthy matter in solution; for Aristotle says in the same treatise that sea-water "has much more body" than drinking-water.[409] Still speaking of spontaneous generation he says a little further on : —

["Whoever would inquire aright should ask: What product in such cases answers to that material principle which in the female is a certain animal excretion,[410] potentially similar to what it came from? That excretion is quickened by the principle derived from the male, which thus perfects the animal. In the present case what should be likened to that excretion, and whence and what is the quickening principle which answers to the principle from the male? Now we must assume that, even in animals which procreate, the heat within the animal [411] separates and concocts, and thus makes out of the nourishment which enters the animal the excretion which is the beginning of the embryo. Such is the case with plants likewise; although in these and in some animals there is no need of the principle imparted by the male, for this they have within and mingled with themselves; whereas in most animals the excretion aforesaid stands in need of that principle. The nourishment of some is water and earth, that of others is derived from water and earth; so that what the heat in animals [412] prepares out of their nourishment, the heat of the season in the circumambient air combines by concoction out of the sea and the earth, and puts together.[413] But so much of the psychical principle as is included or separated within the air [319] constructs and quickens [414] the embryo. In like manner are put together such plants as arise by spontaneous generation." [415]

The doctrine that in sexual generation the semen furnishes soul and generative heat but none of the matter [416] of which the embryo consists, renders logical the view, which Aristotle would seem to hold, that it is soul from the air and generative heat from the sun which in spontaneous generation represent the derivatives from the male. [417]   The presence about us of "the psychical principle," thus diffused, may well seem startling to a modern biologist; but we may remind ourselves that in ancient times many believed the soul to be conveyed by the air into even the higher animals; even into man himself, even man's "understanding" reaching him thus. [418]   Indeed, not only the words "*pneuma*" and "*spiritus*," as we have learned, but also the Greek and Latin words for "soul," viz.: "*psyche*" and "*anima*," meant originally simply "breath."   Let us recall the words of scripture, which seem so vivid to one who watches the change in a new-born child as the first breath is taken: "And the Lord God formed man of the dust of the ground, and breathed into his nostrils the breath of life; and man became a living soul." [419]

That the soul enters with the breath is, however, expressly denied by Aristotle.   Conceding a share of soul to every living thing he points out quite simply that there are animals which do not breathe at all, to say nothing of plants. [420]   Clearly, the doctrine which he rejects would be hard to reconcile with his theory of sexual generation, according to which theory the sensory soul, and in man even the divine intellectual soul, is potential in the semen and imparted thereby to the product of conception. [421]   Indeed, there is a chapter of Aristotle's treatise On Soul in which he even

seems to argue against the presence of soul in the air,
in a polemic directed against those who believe the soul
to be "composed of the elements." [422]   In this polemic
he is the subtle philosopher; but in his statements
about generation he seems more the biologist; for in
these his thought, if not more ripe, appears to be less
concerned with disputation than with phenomena and
the interpretation thereof.

The generation of living things is but generation
still, whether it be sexual or spontaneous; and the
modern student of general physiology may trace further
parallels of thought in Aristotle's account of spontaneous generation and in those words of his about the
semen which Harvey quotes and we have studied.
That living rudiment, spontaneously generated, which
consists of a foam-bubble whose film of earth and water
was formed by the heat of the sun and includes air
charged with generative heat associated with soul —
surely that reminds one of the foamy semen, and of
"the spirits included in the semen and in foaminess,"
and of that within the spirits "which makes semen
generative, the so-called heat," the "nature which is
analogous to the element of the stars," which nature is
derived from the male parent and is associated with the
soul potential in the semen.   In the Greek text of
Aristotle one and the same word, "*pneuma*," is used
to express both the air in the foam-bubbles of spontaneous generation, and the vapor in the foam-bubbles
of the semen.   In translation "*pneuma*" must be
rendered "spirits" in the case of the semen, and the
verbal identity is lost which, by reason of the very
vagueness of the Greek word, helps to mark the parallel-

ism of thought. It is with *pneuma*, spirits, that the
testicles and breasts are swollen at the advent of pu-
berty,[423] according to Aristotle ; and with the presence
of *pneuma* he connects the pleasure of the sexual act.[424]
We have found him laying stress upon the fact that
"the nature of semen is foamy" — that its "generative
medium [ἡ γονή] is foam" : and he tells of the spontaneous generation of certain shellfish in a place where
there is "foamy mud." [425] When he obscurely says
that in the semen "the *pneuma* included in the semen
and in foaminess" [426] is the vehicle of the generative
heat, does not the turn of phrase indicate that Aristotle's
thought is ranging far, that he is thinking not only of
the foam of the semen but of other widely different
kinds of prolific foam as well? Does he not seem to
think that, in general, the power of bringing matter to
life as a new individual dwells typically in a bubble
representing earth, water, and air, and charged with
soul and with generative heat, for the presence of
which the sun is responsible, heat other than that
of elemental fire? [320] It is not fanciful — for Aristotle himself, we remember, has done so incidentally — to connect such speculation with the ancient
myth of Aphrodite, the goddess of love, who sprang
from the foam which had risen upon the sea, about
the immortal genitals of Uranus, which had been
severed and cast therein ; Uranus being the heavens
personified.[427]

Before the time of Aristotle important thinkers had
held the heavenly bodies, and even the heavens themselves, to be fire ; [428] and we have seen that after his
time Cleanthes did the same, simply setting apart the

generative fire from the destructive. Aristotle denied
that the sun is fire, though he could not have denied
that its radiant generative heat produces no different
sensation from that of sterile fire kindled upon earth.
He did not identify the sun's heat with ether, the "body
on high," though he styled the heat of the semen a
"body" analogous to the ether. How then did Aristotle obtain heat from the ethereal sun? The point
is crucial and he met it ; but in so doing he revealed a
very weak place in his towering fabric of speculation.
In his treatise On Heaven, speaking of the heavenly
bodies, he says : —

"The heat and light from these arise from the friction which the
air undergoes by reason of their course. For it is the nature of
motion to fire even wood and stone and steel."

He then speaks of projectiles, and says : —

"These, then, are heated because borne onward in air which becomes fire from the shock of the motion. But each of the bodies
on high is borne onward in its sphere, so that they are not fired ;
while the air, being beneath the sphere of the circling body,[429] is
heated of necessity as this [body] is borne onward, and mainly
where the sun is set in place. Therefore, when the sun approaches
and rises and is above us, heat is generated. Be it said, then, of the
heavenly bodies, that neither are they fiery nor are they borne on
in fire." [430]

In his Meteorology Aristotle boldly says : "The sun,
which is held to be especially hot, appears white, but
not to be like fire." [431]
Hardy thinker as he is, however, Aristotle nowhere
undertakes to tell how the heat of friction between the
air and the circling "first element" on high becomes
generative, as opposed to the heat of friction between

the air and a projectile composed of the lower elements.
As to this the Aristotle who deals with the heavens does
not strike hands with Aristotle the biologist; nor is
light thrown by its author on the Aristotelian passage
quoted by Harvey, in which alone does the generative
heat of animals figure as "the nature which is analogous
to the elements of the stars"; [432] nor yet does the
Aristotelian dictum that "Man and the sun generate
man" [338] remain other than a great truth which awaits
elucidation.

More than nineteen centuries after Aristotle's death
Harvey published the following, in his treatise On
Generation : —

"Thus the sun and man, that is, the sun through man as an instrument, generate. In the same way the Father of all and the
cock generate the egg and the chick derived from the egg; namely,
by means of the perpetual approach and withdrawal of the sun,
which by the will of divine authority, or by fate if you choose, serves
for the generation of all things.

"Our conclusion, then, is that the male, although a prior and more
important efficient cause than the female, is only an instrumental
efficient cause; that he, no less than the female, receives his
fecundity or generative power from the approaching sun; and
that, accordingly, the art and providence which we discern in his
works proceed not from himself but from God." [433]

Two pages farther on Harvey says, again : —

"In fact, what the cock confers upon the egg to make it no
longer a wind-egg but prolific, is the same that is bestowed by the
summer fervor of the sun upon vegetable fruits, that they may
reach maturity, and their seeds, fecundity; and the same that
imparts fecundity to beings that arise spontaneously [434] and that
produces caterpillars out of worms, chrysalides out of caterpillars,
out of chrysalides, butterflies, flies, bees, and the rest." [435]

In a later Exercise of the same treatise Harvey says : —

"As I have said, the product of conception in viviparous creatures is analogous to the seed and fruit of plants; as also is the egg
in the ovipara; in creatures which come into existence spontaneously, the worm; [436] or some bubble of confined moisture [437] pregnant with vital heat. In all of the foregoing exists that which is
the same in all, that in virtue of which they are called with truth
seeds; that, namely, out of which and by which, preëxisting as
matter, artificer, and instrument, every animal is in the first instance made and comes into existence." [438]

Despite emphatic denials of Aristotelian doctrine
which Harvey freely makes in his treatise On Generation, the Aristotelian flavor of the foregoing passages is
obvious. It is not easy to make out from Harvey's
writings the exact nature of his views as to spontaneous
generation. He sometimes seems to assume the truth
thereof; but it is by no means certain that he believed
in it in the same simple sense in which it had been
accepted by Aristotle.[439] Nothing, however, can be
clearer than this : that, though for Harvey the "innate
heat" is not ethereal spirits nor even an analogue of the
ether, but is simply identical with the living blood;
nevertheless, for him as emphatically as for Aristotle
the "heat in animals" which "is not fire and does not
take its origin from fire," derives its origin from the
solar ray.

To Harvey, the lifelong thinker upon the meaning
of the circulation, the prodigious history of generation
was but continued in the history of the blood, with
which he had identified the "innate heat" and which he
saw appear and live, before all other parts, in the minute
first rudiment of the embryo. We have seen him

pondering the cycle wherein unending life is transmitted
from egg to fowl and from fowl to egg beneath the sun's
life-giving rays.   So now shall we see him pondering a
cycle of life wherein, from generation to generation, the
circulating blood takes over and exercises the generative
powers of the semen from which it is derived, and
transmits them in turn to the semen evolved out of
itself.   He says : —

"Further, since we have just seen the study of the semen to be
so difficult; that is to say, the way in which the structure of the
body is built up by the semen with foresight, art, and divine intelligence; why should we not equally admire the excellent nature of
the blood, and make the same reflections upon it as upon the semen?
Especially since the semen itself is made of blood,[40] as is proved
in the case of the egg; and since the whole body is seen not only
to take origin from the blood as from a generative part, but also to
owe its preservation to the same." [41]

To this same theme Harvey returns in his Exercise
On the Innate Heat near the end of his treatise On
Generation, saying : —

"The blood, too, acts in like manner above the powers of the elements, because, when it has come into existence as the first generated part and the innate heat, as is brought to pass in the semen
and spirits, the blood constructs the remaining parts of the whole
body in order; and does so with the highest foresight and understanding,[42] acting to a certain end and as though by some use of
reason.[43]   Surely the blood does not accomplish these things because it is composed of elements and draws its origin from fire, but
because by the grace of plastic power and vegetative soul it is made
the first generated heat and the immediate and fitting instrument
of life." [44]

CHAPTER XII

THE CIRCULATION OF THE BLOOD AND THE CIRCULATION OF THE HEAVENS

THE discoverer of the circulation would have been no fit pupil of Aristotle if he had limited his ken to the microcosm; nor were such limitations common in an age when astrology was not so far out of countenance as now. We have found Harvey discussing "the element of the stars" and reverently affirming the dependence of all life upon the sun as well as upon its Creator. We have found him also, in dealing with the powers of the blood, affirming that "lower and corruptible things are subject to other higher and incorruptible things," and in that connection paraphrasing a passage in which Aristotle deals with "the Cosmos which is about the earth." Of this — that is, of the sum of things between our globe and the moon's sphere — the ancient philosopher says: —

"Of necessity it is conjoined, in a way, with the courses on high, so that its entire power is governed thence; for that which originates motion in everything must be recognized as first cause." [445]

In "the courses on high" the divine living existences of heaven circulated forever, ruling the lower Cosmos as cycle succeeded cycle in endless series and the seasons endlessly recurred. In a few pregnant words Aristotle had dealt with the results of this Cosmic circulation, as follows: —

154

"There is said to be a circle in the affairs both of mankind and of whatever else is possessed of natural motion and is subject to generation and corruption." [446]

It was in Harvey's lifetime that this stupendous circulation of the heavens "and all that is in them" received its death stroke.   Throughout Harvey's years of study at Padua, Galileo had lectured there with great acclaim; and after Harvey's return to London discovery after discovery had followed Galileo's work with the telescope, and had dealt blow after blow to the ancient astronomy.   The trial of Galileo had followed; and he had died in 1642, nine years before the publication of Harvey's work On Generation.   Yet belief in the ancient astronomy died far harder than belief in the ancient physiology of the movement of the blood. The ancient astronomy was based on the evidence of every man's own eyes, and flattered human vanity with the doctrine that the whole universe was centered upon the globe of which the ordained possessor was the creature made in the image of God.   Milton had visited Galileo, famous long before, near Florence in 1638; but in the "Paradise Lost," published in 1667,[447] Milton expressly treated the question between the ancients and the followers of Copernicus as an open one, though Copernicus had died in 1543.   Indeed, we find Harvey himself, seven years after Galileo's death, speaking of "the reason why our knowledge of the heavenly bodies is uncertain and conjectural"; [448] and saying of opponents of the circulation of the blood : "Nor do they find it satisfactory to set up new systems, as in astronomy, unless these explain all the phenomena." [449]

It need not surprise us, therefore, to find Harvey

writing as follows in 1628 in the very act of naming his own great discovery : —

"I beg leave to call this motion circular in the same sense in which Aristotle said that air [450] and rain imitate the circular motion of the bodies on high.[451]   For the earth, when wet and warmed by the sun, gives off vapor; the vapors are borne upward and condensed and, when condensed into rain, descend again and wet the earth.   Thus, too, generation here below and, in like manner, the arising of tempests and meteors result from the circular motion of the sun, his approach and recession." [452]

In 1651, nine years after the death of Galileo, in the last words about the moving blood which Harvey published, he drew a parallel between the circulation of the microcosm and the mighty circulation of the macrocosm. This parallel is drawn just before the end of his final work, his treatise On Generation, in a passage of his Exercise On the Innate Heat, in words which may serve to sum up what has gone before.   These words shall be quoted without further comment and shall bring our present study of Harvey to an end : —

"The following few points should be considered well by every diligent mind, and so the fact becomes established more clearly, that those remarkable virtues which learned men attribute to the spirits and the innate heat are appropriate to the blood alone; to say nothing of what is so wonderfully striking in the egg before aught of the embryo has appeared, and in the perfect and developed embryo also.   To be sure, the blood, considered absolutely and by itself outside the veins and regarded as consisting of elements [453] and as composed of different parts, — some thin and serous, some thick and solidified, — is termed 'cruor' and is possessed of very few virtues, and those obscure.   But the blood, when present within the veins as a part of the body, a generative part, too, and endowed with soul, being the soul's immediate instrument and primary seat — the blood, seeming also to have a share of another diviner body and being suffused with divine heat, certainly acquires extraordinary powers, and is analogous to the element of the stars. As spirits the blood is the hearth, the Vesta,[454] the household deity, the innate heat, the sun of the microcosm, the fire of Plato; [455] not because it shines, burns, and destroys, like common fire, but because it preserves and nourishes and increases its very self by its perpetual wandering motion. Moreover, the blood deserves the name of spirits because, primarily and before all other parts, it abounds in radical moisture, that is, in the final and most immediate form of nourishment; and the same fare wherewith the blood itself is nourished is made ready by it and given out to all other parts while it is coursing perpetually through the entire body. Indeed, the blood nourishes, fosters, and keeps alive all the parts which it constructs and adjoins to itself, even as the heavenly bodies above, especially the sun and moon, impart life to what is below, while they continue in perpetual circulation. Since, therefore, the blood acts beyond the powers of the elements and is potent with those virtues aforesaid, and also is the instrument of the supreme workman, no one ever will give praise enough to its wonderful and divine faculties."[456]

Let us end these studies by picturing to ourselves the memorable figure of the small white-haired man ensconced in one of his favorite nooks on the leads of his brother's house, musing upon the mystery of the circulation, and linking it with that of

> "The shining powers, conspicuous afar
> Against the ether, which to mortals bring
> Winter and summer." [457]

NOTES

[1] In the present paper frequent references will be made to the writings of Harvey, Galen, Aristotle, and Hippocrates. Citations from these authors will be made from the following editions: —

References to Harvey's finished writings will be made to two editions, viz.: The Works of William Harvey, translated from the Latin with a life of the author by R. Willis, M.D., London, 1847, printed for the Sydenham Society, which will here be designated as "Syd."; and Guilielmi Harveii Opera Omnia: A Collegio Medicorum Londinensi Edita: 1766, which will be designated as "Op. Omn." In the preparation of the text the present writer has used these two editions and also the first editions of Exercitatio Anatomica de Motu Cordis et Sanguinis in Animalibus, Frankfort, 1628, and Exercitationes de Generatione Animalium, London, 1651. Willis's translation of passages has been revised, often freely, where the writer has judged this desirable; and sometimes the revision amounts to a fresh translation. References to Harvey's lecture notes will be made to Prelectiones Anatomiæ Universalis by William Harvey, edited with an autotype reproduction of the original by a committee of the Royal College of Physicians, London, 1886.

References to Galen's writings will be made to two editions, viz.: Claudii Galeni Opera Omnia. Editionem curavit C. G. Kühn, Leipsic, 1821–1833, which will be designated by the letters "Kn."; and Œuvres Anatomiques, Physiologíques et Medicáles de Galien, Traduites avec Notes par C. Daremberg, Paris, 1854–1856, which will be cited as "Dar." The former is the recognized working edition of the Greek text of Galen; this is accompanied by a Latin translation, to which is appended a serviceable Latin index. By the pages of this edition the Greek text of Galen is commonly cited. None of the treatises of Galen has been translated into English. Some of those most interesting to physiologists may be read in the above French translation of Daremberg. A critical edition of the Greek text of Galen's treatise On the Doctrines of Hippocrates and Plato, Claudii Galeni de Placitis Hippocratis et Platonis, with an

159

amended Latin translation by Johannes Müller, was published by Teubner, Leipsic, 1874; it will here be cited as "Mül."

References to Aristotle's writings will be made to Aristotelis Opera: Edidit Academia Regia Borussica, Berlin, 1831–1870, which is the commonly cited Greek text. Pages and lines of this edition will always be found in the margin of a modern edition or translation. The following works of Aristotle will be referred to in this paper : —

The Psychology and its appendices, viz.: the so-called "Lesser Works on Natural Things (Parva Naturalia)." English translation by W. A. Hammond, New York, 1902. The two last treatises of the Parva Naturalia have also been translated by W. Ogle, M.D., London, 1897.

The History of Animals. English translation by R. Creswell. Bohn's Classical Library. London, 1878.

On the Parts of Animals. English translation by W. Ogle, M.D., London, 1882.

On the Generation of Animals. There is no English translation. An excellent German translation, with the Greek text, is that by Aubert and Wimmer, Leipsic, 1860.

Physics. There is no English translation; Greek text and German translation by C. Prantl, Leipsic, 1854.

On Heaven: On Generation and Corruption (In the Universe at Large). There is no English translation; Greek text and German translation by C. Prantl, Leipsic, 1857.

Meteorology. There is no English translation; French translation by J. B. St. Hilaire, Paris, 1863.

Besides the foregoing, other treatises by Aristotle may be referred to or cited briefly.

References to the Hippocratic writings will be made to Œuvres Complètes d'Hippocrate, traduction nouvelle, par É. Littré, Paris, 1839–1861, which will be designated as "Lit." This is the standard working edition of the Greek text of the Hippocratic collection, and is the one now usually cited. The accompanying French translation is complete. There is a translation into English of some of the treatises, but it cannot be recommended. A new version of the Greek text is now in slow course of publication by Teubner of Leipsic.

[1] John Aubrey: 'Brief Lives,' Chiefly of Contemporaries, etc. Edited from the Author's Mss. by Andrew Clark; 1898, Vol. I, 300.

[3] **Harvey**: On Generation, Preface, Syd. 152, l. 34 to 153, l. 4; Op. Omn. 168, l. 22–26.

[4] **Galen**: Is Blood Naturally Contained in the Arteries? Kn. Vol. IV, 703–736.

[5] **Harvey**: On Conception, Syd. 575, l. 9–12; Op. Omn. 592, l. 8–11.

[6] **Harvey**: Letter to Hofmann, Syd. 595, l. 6–15; Op. Omn. 635, l. 10–17.

[7] **Harvey**: Letter to Hofmann, Syd. 596, l. 3–7; Op. Omn. 636, l. 1–4.

[8] **Harvey**: Exercise to Riolanus, II, Syd. 122, l. 31 to 123, l. 1; Op. Omn. 122, l. 16–21.

[9] **Harvey**: On the Motion, etc., VIII, Syd. 47, l. 29–33; Op. Omn. 49, l. 28–30.

[10] **Harvey**: On the Motion, etc., IX, Syd. 48, l. 10–14; Op. Omn. 50, l. 8–11.

[11] Plato: Timæus, 70a and b; 77c to 78a; 78e to 79a.

Aristotle: On the Parts of Animals, 668a, 4 to b, 6.

Galen: On the Natural Faculties, Kn. Vol. II, 210–212; **Dar.** Vol. II, 318.

[12] Aristotle: On Sleep and Waking, 456a, 30 to b, 5.

Galen: On the Use of the Parts, etc., Kn. Vol. III, 269–270; **Dar.** Vol. I, 280–282.

[13] Galen: On the Natural Faculties, Kn. Vol. II, 186–189; **Dar.** Vol. II, 306–307.

[14] **Harvey**: On the Motion, etc., Syd. 72, l. 24 to 73, l. 12; Op. Omn. 73, l. 26 to 74, l. 15.

[15] **Harvey**: On the Motion, etc., Syd. 75, l. 9–22; Op. Omn. 76, l. 15–25.

[16] Joannes Riolanus, Filius: Encheiridium Anatomicum et Pathologicum, etc., Paris, 1648, 298, l. 1–4. Harvey's quotation does complete justice to the sense, but is by no means accurate verbally.

[17] **Harvey**: Exercise to Riolanus, I, Syd. 95, l. 4–21; Op. Omn. 97, l. 6–23.

[18] Aselli: De Lactibus, sive Lacteis Venis, etc. Milan, 1627.

[19] John Aubrey: Brief Lives, etc., 1898, Vol. I, 302.

[20] Harvey's venous artery and arterial vein correspond respectively to the pulmonary vein and the pulmonary artery of our nomenclature.

[21] **Harvey**: On the Motion, etc., VI, Syd. 39, l. 29 to 40, l. 15; Op. Omn. 41, l. 20 to 42, l. 10.

[22] Compare Aristotle : History of Animals, 511b, 10–24.

[23] Harvey : On the Motion, etc., XVII, Syd. 85, l. 17–25 ; Op. Omn. 87, l. 5–12.

[24] Aristotle : On Youth and Old Age, On Life and Death, 469b, 6–20.

[25] Aristotle : On Respiration, 473a, 8–10.

[26] Aristotle : On the Generation of Animals, 732a, 18–20.

[27] Aristotle : On Youth and Old Age, On Life and Death, 469a, 28 to 470a, 18.   On Respiration, 474a, 25 to b, 24 ; 478a, 26 to b, 21 ; 480a, 18 to b, 20.

[28] Aristotle : On Respiration, 478a, 21–30.

[29] διὰ τὴν σύναψιν.

[30] Aristotle : History of Animals, 496a, 27–32.

[31] Hippocrates : On the Heart, Lit. Vol. IX, 86 and 90–92.

[32] Hippocrates : On the Heart, Lit. Vol. IX, 86–88.

[33] Galen : On the Use of Respiration, Kn. Vol. IV, 487–493.

[34] ποιότητος.

[35] Galen : Is Blood Naturally Contained in the Arteries? Kn. Vol. IV, 724–725.

[36] Galen : On the Use of Respiration, Kn. Vol. IV, 510.

[37] Galen : On the Use of the Parts, etc., Kn. Vol. III, 412 ; Dar. Vol. I, 381.

[38] Galen : On the Use of the Pulse, Kn. Vol. V, 149–180.

[39] Harvey : On the Motion, etc., Preface, Syd. 9–14 ; Op. Omn. 9–14.

[40] Galen : On the Use of the Parts, etc., Kn. Vol. III, 636–656 ; Dar. Vol. I, 541–552.

[41] Harvey : Prelectiones, 86 right.

[42] Compare Hippocrates : On Flatus, Lit. Vol. VI, 96.

[43] Harvey : Prelectiones, 86 right.

[44] Galen : On the Use of Respiration, Kn. Vol. IV, 470–471.

[45] Harvey : Prelectiones, 86 right.

[46] Aristotle : On Respiration, 473a, 15 to 474a, 24.   Hippocrates : On the Sacred Disease, Lit. Vol. VI, 368 and 372.

[47] Hippocrates : On the Sacred Disease, Lit. Vol. VI, 368.

[48] Passages which justify the statements here made are among those cited in note 140.

[49] Galen : Is Blood Naturally Contained in the Arteries? Kn. Vol. IV, 703–736.

[50] Galen : On the Use of the Parts, etc., Kn. Vol. III, 541–542 ; Dar. Vol. I, 476.

[51] Plato: Timæus, 69c–d. Archer-Hind's Edition, 254, l. 13 to 256, l. 6.

[52] Aristotle: On Soul, 412a, 1 to 415a, 13.

[53] Galen: On the Doctrines of Hippocrates and Plato, Kn. Vol. V, 608.

[54] Galen: On the Use of the Parts, etc., Kn. Vol. III, 696–703; Dar. Vol. I, 575–579. See also Rapp: "Ueber das Wundernetz," Meckel's Archiv für Anatomie und Physiologie, 1827, 1–13.

[55] Galen: On Methods of Treatment, Kn. Vol. X, 839–840.

[56] On the subject of the spirits the following passages of Galen's works should be consulted, viz.: — On the Natural Faculties, Kn. Vol. II, 204, l. 11 to 206, l. 13; Dar. Vol. II, 315, l. 7 to 316, l. 14; Kn. Vol. II, 214, l. 9–16; Dar. Vol. II, 320, l. 2–9. On the Organ of Smell, Kn. Vol. II, 857–886. On the Use of the Parts of the Human Body, Book VI: Kn. Vol. III, 412, l. 6–12; Dar. Vol. I, 381, l. 4–9; Kn. Vol. III, 487, l. 3 to 488, l. 13; Dar. Vol. I, 438, l. 1 to 439, l. 9; Kn. Vol. III, 490, l. 14 to 492, l. 8; Dar. Vol. I, 440, l. 24 to 441, l. 16; Kn. Vol. III, 496, l. 5–16; Dar. Vol. I, 444, l. 6–19. Book VII: Kn. Vol. III, 536–544; Dar. Vol. I, 472–477; Kn. Vol. III, 544–549; Dar. Vol. I, 477–480. Book VIII: Kn. Vol. III, 636–651; Dar. Vol. I, 541–550; Kn. Vol. III, 651–656; Dar. Vol. I, 550–552; Kn. Vol. III, 663; Dar. Vol. I, 557; Kn. Vol. III, 672–673; Dar. Vol. I, 563. Book IX: Kn. Vol. III, 684–691; Dar. Vol. I, 569–572; Kn. Vol. III, 696–703; Dar. Vol. I, 575–579; Kn. Vol. III, 750–751; Dar. Vol. I, 602–603. Book XIV: Kn. Vol. IV, 183, l. 7–10; Dar. Vol. II, 114, l. 23–25. Book XVI: Kn. Vol. IV, 323, l. 2–18; Dar. Vol. II, 189, l. 3–21; Kn. Vol. IV, 333, l. 18 to 335, l. 10; Dar. Vol. II, 195, l. 6–36. Book XVII: Kn. Vol. IV, 349, l. 5–14; Dar. Vol. II, 202, l. 30–38. On the Causes of Respiration, Kn. Vol. IV, 465–469. On the Use of Respiration, Kn. Vol. IV, 470–511. Is Blood Naturally Contained in the Arteries? Kn. Vol. IV, 703–736. On the Use of the Pulse, Kn. Vol. V, 149–180. On the Doctrines of Hippocrates and Plato, Book II: Kn. Vol. V, 281, l. 3–15; Mül. 245, l. 10 to 246, l. 6. Book III: Kn. Vol. V, 355, l. 18 to 356, l. 11; Mül. 325, l. 16 to 326, l. 9. Book VI: Kn. Vol. V, 524, l. 12 to 525, l. 16; Mül. 512, l. 3 to 513, l. 8; Kn. Vol. V, 571, l. 12 to 573, l. 2; Mül. 563, l. 12 to 566, l. 2. Book VII: Kn. Vol. V, 600–611; Mül. 596–608; Kn. Vol. V, 611–617; Mül. 608–615; Kn. Vol. V, 628, l. 8–15; Mül. 626, l. 8–15; Kn. Vol. V, 641, l. 14 to 642, l. 6; Mül. 641, l. 13 to 642, l. 6. Book VIII: Kn. Vol. V, 707, l. 17 to 710, l. 15; Mül. 714, l. 14 to 718, l. 2.

On Methods of Treatment, Book IX: Kn. Vol. X, 635, l. 6 to 636, l. 12. Book XII: Kn. Vol. X, 839, l. 10 to 840, l. 3.

[57] Harvey: Prelectiones, 83 right.

[58] Harvey: Prelectiones, 85 left.

[59] Harvey: Prelectiones, 83 right and 85 left.

[60] Compare R. Columbus: De Re Anatomica. Venice, 1559, 223–224.

[61] Harvey: Prelectiones, 85 left. The last line of page 85 left, as deciphered and printed, reads as follows: "Galenus 7 & p. 8°." It should read, however, "Galenus 7 u.p. 8°." That this is Harvey's brief reference to Galeni Lib. 7, De Usu Partium, Cap. 8, is proved by the text of the Galenic passage thus referred to, viz.: Galen: On the Use of the Parts, etc., Kn. Vol. III, 539–540, Dar. Vol. I, 475.

[62] As no other claimant than Columbus to be the discoverer of the pulmonary transit of the blood was known to Harvey, the question whether Columbus was the true discoverer, or possibly owed the basis of his doctrine to the unfortunate Michael Servetus, need not here be discussed.

[63] Vesalius: De Humani Corporis Fabrica, Basel, 1543; Lib. VI, Cap. II, 589, l. 9–24. Vesalius: Opera Omnia Anatomica et Chirurgica, Leyden, 1725, Tom. I, De Hum. Corp. Fabr. Lib. VI, Cap. 11, 511, l. 11–23; Cap. 15, 519, l. 42–54. Columbus: De Re Anatomica, Lib. VII, 177, l. 17–24.

[64] Aristotle: On the Parts of Animals, 649b, 19–27.

[65] Harvey: Prelectiones, 85 right. Compare closely similar passages in Harvey: On the Motion, etc., Introduction, Syd. 12, l. 9–15; Op. Omn. 12, l. 10–17. Exercise to Riolanus, II, Syd. 116, l. 26–33; Op. Omn. 116, l. 15–20. On Generation, LXXI, Syd. 504, l. 22–28; Op. Omn. 525, l. 23–29.

[66] The decipherer of Harvey's Ms. notes reads "generatur."

[67] Harvey: On the Motion, etc., Introduction, Syd. 18, l. 16–21; Op. Omn. 18, l. 17–21.

[68] Compare Aristotle: On Respiration, 470b, 28 to 471b, 29.

[69] Harvey: Prelectiones, 86 left.

[70] Harvey: On the Motion, etc., Introduction, Syd. 16, l. 23–27; Op. Omn. 16, l. 21–26.

[71] Harvey: On the Motion, etc., Introduction, Syd. 16, l. 28–39; Op. Omn. 16, l. 27 to 17, l. 4.

[72] πνεῦμα.

[73] Aristotle: History of Animals: 496a, 27–32.

[74] Columbus: De Re Anatomica, Lib. VII, 178–180; Lib. XI, 223–224; Lib. XIV, 259 and 261.

[75] Harvey: Prelectiones, 86 left.

[76] Galen: On the Doctrines of Hippocrates and Plato, Kn. Vol. V, 611–617; Mül. 608–615.

[77] Harvey: Prelectiones, 94 right: "*puto: spiritus Nervis non progredi sed Irradiatos et actus fieri unde sensus et motus ut lumen in aere: forsan ut fluxus et refluxus Maris,*" etc.

[78] Harvey: Exercise to Riolanus, II, Syd. 118, l. 9–14; Op. Omn. 117, l. 29–32.

[79] Harvey: Prelectiones, 86 left.

[80] Columbus: De Re Anatomica, Lib. VI, 166–167; Lib. VII, 177–178; Lib. XI, 22.

Harvey: On the Motion, etc., VII, Syd. 41, l. 7–14; Op. Omn. 43, l. 3–9.

[81] Harvey: Exercise to Riolanus, I, Syd. 98, l. 16–23; Op. Omn. 100, l. 21–28.

[82] Harvey: Exercise to Riolanus, II, Syd. 113–121; Op. Omn. 113–121. On Generation, LXXI, Syd. 501–512; Op. Omn. 523–534.

[83] Harvey: On Generation, LXXI, Syd. 502, l. 33–37; Op. Omn. 524, l. 5–7.

[84] Harvey: On Generation, LXXI, Syd. 504, l. 22–31; Op. Omn. 525, l. 25–32.

[85] Harvey: Exercise to Riolanus, II, Syd. 118, l. 32–38; Op. Omn. 118, l. 16–19.

[86] Harvey: Exercise to Riolanus, II, Syd. 119, l. 3–5 and l. 10–17; Op. Omn. 118, l. 26–28 and 118, l. 30 to 119, l. 4.

[87] Harvey: Prelectiones, 86 right.

[88] Harvey: Exercise to Riolanus, II, Syd. 113, l. 28 to 114, l. 19 and 117, l. 35 to 118, l. 9; Op. Omn. 113, l. 22 to 114, l. 14 and 117, l. 19–29.

[89] Harvey: On Generation, LII, Syd. 388, l. 31–32; Op. Omn. 405, l. 14–15.

[90] Harvey: On Generation, LII, Syd. 386, l. 11–12; Op. Omn. 402, l. 24–26.

[91] Harvey: Prelectiones, 87 left.

[92] Galen: On the Doctrines of Hippocrates and Plato, Kn. Vol. V, 571–572; Mül. 563, l. 12 to 565, l. 9.

[93] Harvey: Exercise to Riolanus, II, Syd. 114, l. 26–29; Op. Omn. 114, l. 19–21.

[94] Harvey: Exercise to Riolanus, II, Syd. 114, l. 37–40; Op. Omn. 114, l. 28–31.

[95] Harvey: Exercise to Riolanus, II, Syd. 115, l. 18–21; Op. Omn. 115, l. 12–14.

[96] Harvey: Exercise to Riolanus, II, Syd. 136, l. 19–21; Op. Omn. 136, l. 12–13.

[97] Harvey: On the Motion, etc., XVII, Syd. 77, l. 24–29; Op. Omn. 79, l. 5–9.

[98] See J. C. Dalton: Doctrines of the Circulation, Philadelphia, 1884, 127–128.

[99] Columbus: De Re Anatomica, Lib. XI, 223, l. 11 to 224, l. 8.

[100] Galen: On the Use of the Parts, etc., Kn. Vol. III, 451–452; Dar. Vol. I, 412, l. 5–8.

[101] Harvey: Letter to Slegel, Syd. 597, l. 14–23; Op. Omn. 613, l. 19–27.

[102] Harvey: On Parturition, Syd. 530, l. 3–10 and l. 25–36; Op. Omn. 549, l. 22–27 and 550 l. 11–20.

[103] Harvey: Letter to Hofmann, Syd. 596, l. 3–7; Op. Omn. 636, l. 1–4.

[104] Harvey: Exercise to Riolanus, II, Syd. 123, l. 15–18; Op. Omn. 122, l. 31 to 123, l. 1.

[105] Harvey: On the Motion, etc., IX, Syd. 48, l. 21 to 50, l. 36; Op. Omn. 50, l. 17 to 52, l. 23.

[106] Harvey: Prelectiones, 80 right.

[107] Hippocrates: On Wounds, Lit. Vol. VI, 430.

[108] Hippocrates: Epidemics, Lit. Vol. V, 114–116. Compare Galen's Third Commentary on Epidemics, Kn. Vol. XVII, A., 433, l. 14 to 436, l. 2.

[109] Harvey: Prelectiones, 79 right.

[110] Harvey: Exercise to Riolanus, II, Syd. 140, l. 30–39; Op. Omn. 140, l. 23–31.

[111] Harvey: Exercise to Riolanus, I, Syd. 98, l. 9–23; Op. Omn. 100, l. 14–28.

[112] Hippocrates: On the Heart, Lit. Vol. IX, 84, l. 11–12.

[113] Aristotle: On Youth and Old Age, etc., 469b, 6–20.

[114] Aristotle: On the Parts of Animals, 670a, 23–26.

[115] Galen: On the Use of Respiration, Kn. Vol. IV, 505, l. 15 to 506, l. 5.

[116] Harvey: On the Motion, etc., VIII, Syd. 46, l. 34 to 47, l. 16; Op. Omn. 49, l. 3–19.

[117] Aristotle: On Respiration; On the Parts of Animals, Books

II and III; and elsewhere. This reference is by Harvey himself.

[118] Aristotle: On the Parts of Animals, Book II. This reference is by Harvey himself.

[119] Harvey: On the Motion, etc., XV, Syd. 68, l. 19 to 69, l. 17; Op. Omn. 69, l. 22 to 70, l. 18.

[120] Harvey: On the Motion, etc., XV, Syd. 70, l. 17–25; Op. Omn. 71, l. 22–29.

[121] Harvey: On the Motion, etc., XVI, Syd. 72, l. 8–11; Op. Omn. 73, l. 13–16.

[122] Harvey: On the Motion, etc., XVII, Syd. 83, l. 9–27; Op. Omn. 84, l. 31 to 85, l. 14.

[123] Hippocrates: On the Nature of the Child, Lit. Vol. VII, 530, l. 3–19.

[124] Aristotle: History of Animals, 561a, 4 to 562b, 2.

[125] Harvey: On the Motion, etc., XVII, Syd. 76, l. 3–10; Op. Omn. 77, l. 14–20. On Generation, XVII, Syd. 235, l. 21–26; Op. Omn. 249, l. 9–13.

[126] Harvey: On the Motion, etc., IV, Syd. 30, l. 14–18 and 30, l. 31 to 31, l. 4; Op. Omn. 32, l. 8–10 and 32, l. 22–30.

[127] Aristotle: On the Parts of Animals, 666a, 8–13.

[128] *Principium.*

[129] Harvey: On the Motion, etc., XVI, Syd. 74, l. 4–15; Op. Omn. 75, l. 9–19.

[130] It would be natural to conjecture that this Aristotelian slighting of spirits derived from the air, taken in connection with Aristotle's exaltation of the vital innate heat, may have had much weight with Harvey, who, although he used the word "spirits" freely, insisted that the blood and the spirits are one. But in this matter the Aristotelian precedent cannot have had the same force for Harvey that it would have for us, because he believed Aristotle to be the author of two treatises in which the spirits are expressly treated, not only as entities, but as entities of great physiological importance, though their relations with the outer air are neglected in one of the treatises and quite obscurely dealt with in the other. (See Harvey: On the Motion, etc., IV, Syd. 29, l. 16–25; Op. Omn. 31, l. 8–16. Do., VI, Syd. 38, l. 7–12; Op. Omn. 40, l. 2–5.) Indeed, Harvey in one of his references to Aristotle directly affirmed that the philosopher had believed in "motor spirits" within the animal body. (See Harvey: On the Motion, etc., XVII, Syd. 81, l. 8–12; Op. Omn. 82, l. 31 to 83, l. 3. Compare [Pseudo-] Aris-

totle: On Spirits, 485a, 5–8; and the Latin translation of the same "by an unknown interpreter," 249b, 13–18.) The two treatises in question are entitled, respectively, "On the Motion of Animals" and "On Spirits," and have been attributed to Aristotle and habitually printed among his works, both before and since the time of Harvey. Modern criticism, however, has made it clear that neither treatise is a genuine work of Aristotle. It is especially plain that the treatise "On Spirits" is by another hand and of another school; among other reasons, because the author declares the skin to be supplied with blood by the veins, and with spirits by accompanying vessels which he calls "arteries." In this treatise the maintenance of the spirits by respiration is discussed, but left uncertain (483b, 15–19). It is but fair to the criticism of Harvey's time to note that, glaringly at variance as the undoubted works of Aristotle are with the treatise "On Spirits," the latter was pronounced genuine, in 1839, by so eminent a scholar as É. Littré, in his "Œuvres d' Hippocrate," etc., Vol. I, 203. Reasons why the treatises in question are not by Aristotle, are given at length in the essay in Latin by V. Rose, entitled "De Aristotelis Librorum Ordine et Auctoritate Commentatio," Berlin, 1854, 162–171, and at the end of 174.

[131] Compare the Iliad, Book XXI, 441.

[132] ἐν τούτῳ γὰρ ἡ φύσις ἐμπεπύρευκεν αὐτήν. Aristotle: On Respiration, 474b, 10–13.

[133] Aristotle: On Youth and Old Age, etc., 469a, 11–12 and 17–20.

[134] Plato: Timæus, 70a–b and 77d–e.

[135] κίνησις.

[136] νεῦρα.

[137] Aristotle: On the Parts of Animals, 666b, 11–16.

[138] Harvey: On the Motion, etc., XVII, Syd. 81, l. 12–19; Op. Omn. 83, l. 3–8.

[139] Harvey: On Generation, XI, Syd. 207, l. 33–35; Op. Omn. 220, l. 26–28.

[140] The foregoing statements and summaries of Aristotelian doctrine are based upon the following portions of Aristotle's works: Meteorology, 366b, 2 to 367a, 3. On Soul, 413a, 11 to 415a, 13; 416a, 9 to b, 31; 426b, 8 to 427a, 16; 429a, 10 to 430a, 9. The following five titles are of treatises among the Parva Naturalia: On Sensation and the Sensible, 438b, 24 to 439a, 5; On Sleep and Waking, 455a, 4 to 458a, 32; On Dreams, 461b, 11–15; On Youth and Old Age, and On Life and Death, the whole treatise; On Res-

piration, 473a, 9–10; 475a, 25 to b, 24; 478a, 11 to b, 21; 479a, 29 to b, 7; 479b, 17 to 480b, 20. History of Animals, 496a, 4 to 497b, 2; 512b, 12 to 515b, 26; 535a, 26 to 536a, 4; 561a, 4 to 562b, 2. Of the History of Animals Book X is clearly spurious; see V. Rose: "De Aristotelis Librorum Ordine et Auctoritate Commentatio," 171–174. Book VII is very probably spurious; see "Aristotelis Thierkunde, etc.," Aubert and Wimmer, 1868, Vol. I, 7–11. On the Parts of Animals, 647b, 29 to 648a, 13; 652b, 1–33; 659b, 13–19; 665a, 28 to 669b, 12; 670a, 23–27; 672a, 22 to b, 7; 677b, 36 to 678a, 3; 678b, 2–4; 689a, 29–31; 697a, 26–29. On the Generation of Animals, 718a, 2–4; 728a, 9–11; 723a, 18–20; 735b, 32 to 736a, 9; 736a, 24 to 737b, 7; 737b, 27 to 738a, 9; 739b, 22–23; 740b, 2 to 741a, 5; 741b, 25 to 742a, 8; 743a, 3 to b, 29; 743b, 35 to 744a, 14; 744a, 26–31; 751b, 6; 752a, 1–4; 755a, 10–25; 762b, 6–9; 766a, 33 to b, 1; 768b, 15–36; 772a, 23–25; 781a, 14 to b, 29; 783b, 29–32; 789b, 7–12. Politics, 1336a, 34–39.

[141] Hippocrates: On the Heart, Lit. Vol. IX, 86–92.

[142] Galen: On the Doctrines of Hippocrates and Plato, Kn. Voi. V, 547–563; Mül. 537, l. 15 to 555, l. 11.

[143] The extant works of Aretæus the Cappadocian; edited and translated by Francis Adams. London, printed for the Sydenham Society, 1856. Therapeutics of Acute Diseases, Book II, Chapter 6, [Greek text] 190; [English translation] 440–441; Chapter 7, [Greek text] 193; [translation] 443.

[144] Hippocrates: On Nourishment, Lit. Vol. IX, 110. Galen: Commentary IV on the foregoing, Kn. Vol. XV, 388–392; On the Doctrines of Hippocrates and Plato, Kn. Vol. V, 529, 531–532 and 577–578; Mül. 517, l. 7–15, 520, l. 2 to 521, l. 4, 570–571.

[145] Galen: On the Use of the Parts, etc., Kn. Vol. III, 451, l. 16 to 452, l. 2; Dar. Vol. I, 412, l. 5–8.

[146] Among Galen's numerous works the following are the treatises and parts of treatises which are most important for a student of Galen's doctrines regarding the movement of the blood. A title quoted without further specification indicates a treatise in one book only, the whole of which should be read. Where no chapters of a book are specified the whole book should be read. The order is that of Kühn's edition: On the Natural Faculties, Book III, chapters 13–15, Kn. Vol. II, Dar. Vol. II. On Anatomical Manipulations, Book VII, chapters 4, 14, 15, 16; Book VIII, chapter 8, Kn. Vol. II. On the Dissection of the Veins and Arteries, chapters 1, 2, 8, 9, Kn. Vol. II. On the Use of the Parts of the Human Body,

Books IV, VI, VII, IX, Kn. Vol. II, Dar. Vol. I, Book XVI, Kn. Vol. IV, Dar. Vol. II. On the Causes of Respiration, Kn. Vol. IV. On the Use of Respiration, Kn. Vol. IV. Is Blood Naturally Contained in the Arteries? Kn. Vol. IV. On the Use of the Pulse, Kn. Vol. V. On the Doctrines of Hippocrates and Plato, Book I, chapter 7, Book II, chapter 8, Book III, chapter 8, Book VI, Book VII, chapter 3, Kn. Vol. V. On the Causes of Disease, chapter 3, Kn. Vol. VII. On the Different Kinds of Pulse, Book IV, chapters 2, 6, 17, Kn. Vol. VIII. On the Causes of the Pulse, Book I, chapters 3, 4, Book II, chapter 15, Kn. Vol. IX. On Prognosis by the Pulse, Book II, chapter 1, Kn. Vol. IX. On Methods of Treatment, Book VIII, chapter 5, Book IX, chapter 10, Book XII, chapter 5, Kn. Vol. X. Commentaries on the Book on Nourishment of Hippocrates, Commentary III, chapters 8, 10, 23, Commentary IV, chapters 4, 6, Kn. Vol. XV. Commentaries on the Book on the Humors of Hippocrates, Commentary III, chapter 31, Kn. Vol. XVI. Commentaries on the Sixth Book of Hippocrates on Epidemic Diseases, Commentary VI, chapters 1–3, Kn. Vol. XVII, Pars II.

[147] For the views of Columbus see his book: De Re Anatomica, Lib. VI, VII, XI, cap. 1, 2, 4; XII and XIII.

[148] Columbus: De Re Anatomica, Lib. VII, 180, l. 1–6.

[149] Harvey: Prelectiones, 33 and 35 right; 74 and 75 left. On the Motion, etc., XVI, Syd. 73, l. 12–17 and l. 24–28; Op. Omn. 74, l. 15–19 and l. 24–28; Do., XVIII, Syd. 83, l. 9–27; Op. Omn. 84, l. 31 to 85, l. 14. On Generation, LIII, Syd. 392, l. 14 to 393, l. 5; Op. Omn. 409, l. 13 to 410, l. 5; Do., LX, Syd. 452, l. 20–28; Op. Omn. 472, l. 1–7. On Uterine Membranes and Humours, Syd. 568, l. 8–27; Op. Omn. 587, l. 19 to 588, l. 5.

[150] Harvey: On the Motion, etc., Syd. 32, l. 39 to 33, l. 31; Op. Omn. 34, l. 24 to 35, l. 19. In Galen's book, from which Harvey here quotes, the quoted passage is preceded by a corrected statement of the mechanics of the valves of the heart, and a declaration that their mechanics were unknown to Erasistratus. Then follow these words: —

"If this be so, O followers of Erasistratus, let us omit all else and consider only what is in controversy. As to the vena cava, which conveys blood from the liver into the heart, in which of two ways are its membranes [i.e. the segments of the tricuspid valve] inserted: do they extend from the interior [of the ventricle] outward, or contrariwise, from without inward? But perhaps this is of no great moment!"

The preceding words are immediately followed by the words quoted by Harvey. The context shows that the phrase "from without inward" indicates the true insertion of the "membranes" of the tricuspid valve, according to both Galen and the facts. Harvey himself refers his quotation from Galen to the treatise "On the Doctrines of Hippocrates and Plato, Book VI." It is from chapter 6 of that book. The Latin text quoted by Harvey, and that from which the quotation in this note has been translated, may be found in the Ninth Juntine Edition of Galen's works, consisting of Latin translations by various hands. This edition was published in Venice in 1625, three years before the publication of Harvey's treatise. The title of the edition is: Galeni Opera ex Nona Juntarum Editione, etc. Venetiis, apud Juntas, MDCXXV, Cum privilegiis. The passage quoted in this note is: "Prima classis," folio 264 D, l. 53–56. Harvey's quotation is: folio 264 D, l. 56 to folio 264 (verso) E, l. 3. The Greek text of the passage quoted in this note is to be found in Kn. Vol. V, 550, l. 9–15; Mül. 541, l. 4–9. The Greek text of Harvey's quotation is in Kn. Vol. V, 550, l. 15 to 551, l. 6; Mül. 541, l. 10 to 542, l. 2. The Latin rendering printed in the Juntine edition gives the true meaning of the Greek text, but in a rather lumbering fashion.

[151] The transit of the blood from the right to the left ventricle.

[152] The Galenic work entitled: "Is Blood Naturally Contained in the Arteries?" Kn. Vol. IV, 703–736.

[153] Harvey: On the Motion, etc., V, Syd. 32, l. 39 to 34, l. 22; Op. Omn. 32, l. 24 to 36, l. 15. The second Galenic passage above, which refers to the origin and contents of the arteries and to the aortic valves, is printed in italics and with quotation marks in the first edition of Harvey's treatise, and Harvey's own words regarding this passage seem to mean that it is a verbal quotation from Galen. But neither in Galen's treatise entitled "Is Blood Naturally Contained in the Arteries?" nor in the sixth book of his treatise On the Doctrines of Hippocrates and Plato, does more than the last part of this seeming quotation occur. The rest appears to be merely a sound statement by Harvey of Galenic doctrines, for which abundant authority can be found in the two treatises aforesaid. See especially for the origin of the arteries: On the Doctrines of Hippocrates and Plato, Book VI, chapter 3, Kn. Vol. V, 524, l. 13 to 525, l. 3; Mül. 512, l. 4–13; and for the contents of the arteries: chapter 4, Kn. Vol. V, 537, l. 1–7; Mül. 526, l. 1–7; and chapter 8, Kn. Vol. V, 572, l. 12 to 573, l. 11; Mül. 565, l. 10

to 566, l. 12. Of the words relating to the aortic valves, the first part is a statement justified by the words which occur in the Ninth Juntine edition of Galen's works, Classis I, folio 264C, l. 41–43 and D, l. 49–53. But the last part of the passage aforesaid is a verbal quotation of words on folio 264 verso F, l. 9–11. This passage relating to the valves is all in Galen's treatise On the Doctrines of Hippocrates and Plato, Book VI, chapter 6. The Greek text may be found as follows: Kn. Vol. V, 549, l. 3–8, 549, l. 18 to 550, l. 6, 552, l. 1–3; Mül. 539, l. 10 to 540, l. 1, 540, l. 11 to 541, l. 1, 543, l. 1–3.

[154] Harvey: Letter to Slegel, Syd. 598, l. 21–23; Op. Omn. 614, l. 29–32.

[155] Aristotle: On Soul, 405b, 1–8.

[156] Harvey: Prelectiones, 80 right. Compare pp. 42–46 of this paper.

[157] Harvey: Prelectiones, 79 right.

[158] That is, one may suppose, after development *in utero* has begun.

[159] *Anima.*

[160] Harvey: Prelectiones, 33 left.

[161] Harvey: Prelectiones, 75 left.

[162] Harvey: Prelectiones, 76 right.

[163] *Non propria ratione.*

[164] *Sanguinis multitudine.*

[165] *Pullulare.*

[166] The two words "household shrine" represent the one word "lar."

[167] Harvey: Prelectiones, 73 left. In the photograph of folio 73 left of Harvey's note-book, the 16th line of text consists, as translated, of the words "Is there only a drop of blood in the auricles?" This line has the appearance of an interlineation. If it be really such, the words which follow it to the end of the passage were meant, when jotted down, to refer to the heart and not to "a drop of blood."

[168] *Rationem.* Compare Harvey: On Generation, LXXI, Syd. 507, l. 16–26; Op. Omn. 528, l. 21–29.

[169] Harvey: Exercise to Riolanus, II, Syd. 136, l. 37 to 137, l. 17; Op. Omn. 136, l. 25 to 137, l. 9.

[170] Harvey: On Generation, Introduction, Syd. 167, l. 2–5; Op. Omn. 180, l. 23–26.

[171] Harvey: On Generation, XIV, Syd. 226, l. 38 to 227, l. 16; Op. Omn. 240, l. 22 to 241, l. 3.

[172] *Animalis.*

[173] Harvey: On Generation, XLVI, Syd. 341, l. 25–37; Op. Omn. 357, l. 5–15.

[174] That is, the mammalian embryo.

[175] Harvey: On Generation, LIII, Syd, 392, l. 1–13; Op. Omn. 409, l. 1–12.

[176] Harvey: On the Motion, etc., Dedication to the King, Syd. 3, l. 2–3; Op. Omn. 3, l. 2. On the Motion, etc., VIII, Syd. 47, l. 7–9; Op. Omn. 49, l. 13–14.

[177] *Idque non solum in ovo, sed in omni fœtu, animaliumque conceptu primo contingere, mox palam fiet.* Harvey: On Generation, *Editio princeps,* 149, l. 33–35. In the Opera Omnia, 390, l. 1–3, a comma has been erroneously placed between "*conceptu*" and "*primo*"; the latter word qualifies "*conceptu,*" not "*contingere.*" Compare Op. Omn. 391, l. 4: *in primis animalium conceptibus.*

[178] *In primis animalium conceptibus.*

[179] Harvey: On Generation, LI, Syd. 373, l. 35 to 374, l. 27 and 374, l. 36 to 375, l. 8; Op. Omn. 389, l. 28 to 390, l. 22 and 390, l. 30 to 391, l. 8.

[180] Harvey: Exercise to Riolanus, II, Syd. 137, l. 2–4 and 138, l. 12–13; Op. Omn. 136, l. 29–30 and 138, l. 6–7.

[181] Milton: Areopagitica, edited with introduction and notes by J. W. Hales, Oxford, 1874, 38.

[182] The "point" is the embryonic heart, to which in its earliest visible state the name of "*punctum saliens,*" *i.e.,* "leaping point," had been given, this technical term having been coined no doubt out of expressions used by Aristotle in speaking of the living rudimentary heart as seen with the naked eye in the hen's egg and in mammalian abortions. Compare Aristotle: History of Animals, 561a, 6–17; On the Parts of Animals, 665a, 33 to b, 2.

[183] Presumably the terminal sinus of modern embryology.

[184] The fourth day of incubation.

[185] *Per totum colliquamentum.* For Harvey's account of this clear liquid see On Generation, XVI, Syd. 232, l. 15 to 234, l. 31; Op. Omn. 246, l. 4 to 248, l. 17.

[186] Aristotle: History of Animals, Book VI, chapter 3. This reference is Harvey's own. Aristotle's words are πόροι φλεβικοί (561a, 13), which are given by Harvey as "*meatus venales.*"

[187] Harvey: On Generation, XVII, Syd. 237, l. 16 to 238, l. 12 and 238, l. 25–35; Op. Omn. 251, l. 6 to 252, l. 3 and 252, l. 15–22.

[188] Harvey: On Generation, XIX, Syd. 252, l. 1 and l. 9–11; Op. Omn. 266, l. 3 and l. 11–13.

[189] Harvey: On Generation, XVI, Syd. 415, l. 22–24; Op. Omn. 433, l. 22–24.

[190] Harvey: On Generation, LVI, Syd. 415, l. 32–38; Op. Omn. 433, l. 31 to 434, l. 4.

[191] Harvey: On the Motion, etc., IV, Syd. 30, l. 14–22; Op. Omn. 32, l. 8–14.

[192] Harvey: On Generation, LI, Syd. 373, l. 35 to 374, l. 27; Op. Omn. 389, l. 28 to 390, l. 22.

[193] ἡ ἀρχή.

[194] ἀλλὰ καὶ περὶ τὴν τελευτήν.

[195] ὥσπερ τῆς φύσεως διαυλοδρομούσης καὶ ἀνελιττομένης ἐπὶ τὴν ἀρχὴν ὅθεν ἦλθεν.

[196] Aristotle: On the Generation of Animals, 741b, 15–24.

[197] In his lecture notes Harvey, in dealing with the heart, speaks of the right auricle as "the last to pulsate." Prelectiones, 74 right, l. 17.

[198] Harvey: On the Motion, etc., IV, Syd. 28, l. 23–34 and 29, l. 6–16; Op. Omn. 30, l. 13–24 and 31, l. 1–8.

[199] Leviticus XVII, 11 and 14 — Harvey's own reference.

[200] Harvey: On Generation, LI, Syd. 376, l. 14 to 377, l. 2 ; Op. Omn. 392, l. 15 to 393, l. 6.

[201] Harvey: On Generation, XVII, Syd. 239, l. 32 to 240, l. 7; Op. Omn. 253, l. 19–31.

[202] Harvey: On the Motion, etc., IV, Syd. 28, l. 15–21; Op. Omn. 30, l. 7–12.

[203] Harvey: On Generation, LI, Syd. 374, l. 28–35; Op. Omn. 390, l. 23–29. Compare: On the Motion, etc., XVII, Syd. 76, l. 11–29; Op. Omn. 77, l. 21 to 78, l. 9.

[204] Harvey: Exercise to Riolanus, II, Syd. 122, l. 31 to 123, l. 18, 124, l. 28–37, 130, l. 29 to 132, l. 25; Op. Omn. 122, l. 16 to 123, l. 2, 124, l. 11–17, 130, l. 15 to 132, l. 17.   On Generation, LXXI, Syd. 503, l. 15–18; Op. Omn. 524, l. 21–24.   Letter to Morison, Syd. 604, l. 13–19; Op. Omn. 620, l. 24 to 621, l. 3.

[205] Harvey: Exercise to Riolanus, II, Syd. 137, l. 15–16; Op. Omn. 137, l. 7–9.

[206] Harvey: Exercise to Riolanus, II, Syd. 136, l. 37 to 138, l. 16; Op. Omn. 136, l. 25 to 138, l. 10.

[207] Harvey: On Generation, LI, Syd. 375, l. 8–39; Op. Omn. 391, l. 9 to 392, l. 2.

208 ἡ ζύμη.

209 πνευματουμένου.

210 Aristotle: On the Generation of Animals, 755a, 18–21.

211 ζέσις.

212 πνευματουμένου.

213 Aristotle: On Respiration, 479b, 26–27 and 30–32.

214 πρὸς τὸν ἔσχατον χιτῶνα.

215 ἀναθυμιασις.

216 διὰ τὸ ἠρτῆσθαι ἐκ τῆς καρδίας.

217 ὅτε.

218 πήδησις, i.e., the "palpitation" of modern medicine.

219 πνευμάτωσις.

220 Aristotle: On Respiration, 480a, 2–15.

221 Aristotle: History of Animals, 521a, 6–7.

222 Galen: On Local Affections, Kn. Vol. VIII, 429, l. 10–12; Dar. Vol. II, 693, l. 35–37. Plutarch: On the Opinions of the Philosophers, Book IV, chapter 22, Diels: Doxographi Graeci, Berlin, 1879, 412, l. 7–9.

223 Galen: On the Motion of the Muscles, Kn. Vol. IV, 367, l. 1–3 and 382, l. 14 to 383, l. 2; Dar. Vol. II, 321, l. 1–3 and 330, l. 3–8.

224 Harvey: On the Motion, etc., XVII, Syd. 81, l. 20–31 and 82, l. 29 to 83, l. 8; Op. Omn. 83, l. 9–18 and 84, l. 15–30.

225 Harvey: Exercise to Riolanus, II, Syd. 137, l. 17–22; Op. Omn. 137, l. 27–32.

226 *Cuius vero rei gratia? Aristotelis. Nullius sed passio ut in pulte ebulliente WH sed vulneratum non flatum sed sanguinem Emittit.* Harvey: Prelectiones, 79 right.

227 *Non ab attractione aliqua.*

228 Harvey: Exercise to Riolanus, II, Syd. 140, l. 15–29; Op. Omn. 140, l. 11–22.

229 Harvey: Letter to Morison, Syd. 604, l. 22–33; Op. Omn. 621, l. 6–15.

230 Harvey: Exercise to Riolanus, II, Syd. 132, l. 26 to 133, l. 14; Op. Omn. 132, l. 18 to 133, l. 11.

231 Harvey: Exercise to Riolanus, II, Syd. 113, l. 24–25; Op. Omn. 113, l. 19–20.

232 Harvey: On the Motion, etc., XVII, Syd. 80, l. 32; Op. Omn. 82, l. 15–16.

233 Compare Harvey: Exercise to Riolanus, II, Syd. 122, l. 19–28; Op. Omn. 122, l. 8–14.

[224] Harvey: On the Motion, etc., IV, Syd. 27, l. 25–27; Op. Omn. 29, l. 12–14.

[225] *Ad constitutionem suam.* Harvey: On the Motion, etc., XVII, Syd. 80, l. 39 to 81, l. 3; Op. Omn. 82, l. 22–26.

[226] Harvey: Prelectiones, 79 left, l. 19 and 80 left, l. 8–10; Columbus: De Re Anatomica, Lib. XI, 223, l. 37–39 and 224, l. 16–21.

[227] Harvey: Exercise to Riolanus, II, Syd. 132, l. 11–15; Op. Omn. 132, l. 4–7.

[228] *Quia non pulsant. sed potius attrahi.* The jotting would seem to leave the verb "*videntur*," or the like, to be understood. Harvey: Prelectiones, 80 left, l. 8–13.

[229] *Eodem tempore tactu sentitur pulsus Arteriae quasi attrahitur vena cava.* Harvey: Prelectiones, 77 right, l. 11–12.

[230] Harvey: On the Motion, etc., Syd. 21, l. 23–27; Op. Omn. 23, l. 16–19. Compare Exercise to Riolanus, II, Syd. 139, l. 26 to 140, l. 29; Op. Omn. 139, l. 21 to 140, l. 22.

[231] *Auriculae pulsant post emotum cor sanguinis multitudine.* Harvey: Prelectiones, 73 left, l. 10.

[232] Harvey: Prelectiones, 77 right, l. 15.

[233] *Quorum radicale humidum glutinosum magis, aut pingue, et lentum est, et non ita facile dissolubile.*

[234] Harvey: On the Motion, etc., IV, Syd. 28, l. 4–14; Op. Omn. 29, l. 29 to 30, l. 6.

[235] Harvey: Exercise to Riolanus, II, Syd. 138, l. 9–11; Op. Omn. 138, l. 4–6.

[236] Galen: On Anatomical Manipulations, Kn. Vol. II, 614, l. 8–11. On the Doctrines of Hippocrates and Plato, Kn. Vol. V, 238, l. 7 to 239, l. 1; Mül. 198, l. 4–16.

[237] Cicero: On the Nature of the Gods, Müller, Leipsic, 1903, 55, l. 20–22. Harvey says in his lecture notes: "*Item* Cicero [has] much about the use of the parts in De Natura Deorum libro 2°." Prelectiones, 98 left, l. 25.

[238] Vesalius: De Humani Corporis Fabrica, Lib. VI, cap. 8, 584, l. 53–57.

[239] Harvey: On the Motion, etc., Syd. 53, l. 26 to 54, l. 15; Op. Omn. 55, l. 21 to 56, l. 11.

[240] For the references to Galileo Galilei, Evangelista Torricelli and Blaise Pascal, see J. C. Poggendorff, Geschichte der Physik, Leipsic, 1879, 251–255, 319–325 and 328–334.

[241] S. Hales: Statical Essays, containing Hæmastaticks, etc. Vol. II, London, 1733. Preface, pp. xvii, l. 13 to xviii, l. 22 and

Experiment III, 13, l. 13 to 17, l. 3. See also P. M. Dawson: The Biography of Stephen Hales, D.D., F.R.S., Johns Hopkins Hospital Bulletin, Vol. XV, No. 159, June, 1904, 185–192. Stephen Hales the Physiologist, Do., Vol. XV, Nos. 160–161, July–August, 1904, 232–237.

[252] Harvey: Exercise to Riolanus, II, Syd. 134, l. 7–16; Op. Omn. 134, l. 8–15.

[253] Harvey: Exercise to Riolanus, II, Syd. 135, l. 12–16; Op. Omn. 135, l. 11–15.

[254] Harvey: Exercise to Riolanus, I, Syd. 93, l. 37 to 94, l. 5; Op. Omn. 95, l. 29 to 96, l. 4.

[255] Harvey: Letter to Slegel, Syd. 598, l. 36 to 602, l. 34; Op. Omn. 615, l. 10 to 619, l. 7.

[256] *Cacochymica.*

[257] Harvey: Exercise to Riolanus, II, Syd. 124, l. 5–10; Op. Omn. 123, l. 25–29.

[258] Harvey: Exercise to Riolanus, II, Syd. 122, l. 9–12; Op. Omn. 122, l. 1–3.

[259] Harvey: Letter to Slegel, Syd. 602, l. 7–10; Op. Omn. 618, l. 18–21.

[260] *Quasi versus principium.*

[261] *Et contra spontaneum moveatur.*

[262] Harvey: On the Motion, etc., XV, Syd. 70, l. 33 to 71, l. 11; Op. Omn. 72, l. 4–17.

[263] *Lacuna.*

[264] *Declinante sponte sanguine et, venarum motu, compresso ad centrum.* Harvey: On the Motion, etc., IV, Syd. 27, l. 33–35; Op. Omn. 29, l. 19–21.

[265] Malpighi: Letter II Regarding the Lungs, Bologna, 1661. Marcelli Malpighii Opera Omnia, Leyden, 1687, Vol. II, 328.

[266] Harvey: Exercise to Riolanus, I, Syd. 96, l. 37 to 97, l. 13; Op. Omn. 99, l. 2–15. The term "circulatory vessels" is one repeated by Harvey from Riolanus, whose views he is here refuting. Riolanus speaks of the region outside the liver, to which the branches of the portal vein are distributed, as the "first region." The "second and third regions" appear to comprise all the rest of the body. See Harvey: Exercise to Riolanus, I, Syd. 90, l. 30 to 91, l. 23; Op. Omn. 92, l. 21 to 93, l. 18. See also Joannes Riolanus, Filius: Encheiridium Anatomicum et Pathologicum, 154, l. 1–13; 155, l. 17 to 156, l. 17; 297, l. 7–17.

[267] *Quibus absorptus et exhaustus traducitur.* Harvey: Exercise

to Riolanus, II, Syd. 133, l. 30–39; Op. Omn. 133, l. 25 to 134, l. 1.

[268] *In sinistri ventriculi locum.*   Harvey: On the Motion, etc., VII, Syd. 45, l. 5–9; Op. Omn. 47, l. 7–10.

[269] Harvey: Exercise to Riolanus, II, Syd. 133, l. 3–6; Op. Omn. 132, l. 30 to 133, l. 2.

[270] Harvey: Prelectiones, 86 left, l. 30–32.

[271] Harvey: Prelectiones, 33 left, l. 31.

[272] Shakspere: Hamlet, Act I, Scene IV, l. 70–73.

[273] αὕτη γὰρ οὐσία ὀφθαλμοῦ ἡ κατὰ τὸν λόγον.

[274] κίνησις.   Cf. p. 52.

[275] δύναμις.

[276] ὅτι ἐστὶν ἡ ψυχὴ τῶν εἰρημένων τούτων ἀρχὴ καὶ τούτοις ὥρισται.

[277] θρεπτικῷ, αἰσθητικῷ, διανοητικῷ, κινήσει.

[278] The foregoing passages from Aristotle's treatise On Soul occur respectively as follows: 412a, 14–15; 414a, 12–14; 412b, 18–22; 413a, 26; 413a, 31; 413a, 20–26; 413a, 31 to b, 16.

[279] οὐθὲν γὰρ αὐτοῦ τῇ ἐνεργείᾳ κοινωνεῖ [σωματικὴ ἐνέργεια].

[280] Aristotle: On the Generation of Animals, 736a, 24 to 737b, 7. The quoted passage is 736b, 28–29.   Compare On Soul, 413b, 24–29.

It was not Greek philosophy alone in which in ancient times the word corresponding to "soul" was used in a wider sense than that of the quotation from "Hamlet."   In the English Authorized Version of the Old Testament, first published in 1611, we read in Genesis II, 7: "Man became a living soul."   The reading is the same in the Revised Version of 1885.   In Genesis I, 30, we read in both versions: "And to every beast of the earth, and to every fowl of the air, and to every thing that creepeth upon the earth, wherein *there is* life, I have given every green herb for meat."   In both versions it is noted in the margin that the expression translated by the single English word "life" is, in the Hebrew, "a living soul." Accordingly we find this Hebrew expression of Genesis I, 30, rendered "a soul of life" — ψυχὴν ζωῆς, — in the ancient translation of the Old Testament into Greek, known as the "Septuagint," which was probably completed less than two hundred years after the death of Aristotle and more than one hundred and fifty years before the Christian era.   In the early Latin translation of the Scriptures which was finished in A.D. 405, and is largely embodied in the "Vulgate" of to-day, we read in the same verse — Genesis I, 30, "*anima viviens*" — "a living soul."   In Genesis II, 7, where the reference is to man himself and the English Bible reads "a living soul," the Vulgate reads "*animam viventem*," using the same Latin words as for the lower creatures of I, 30. In like manner the Septuagint reads in Genesis II, 7, ψυχὴν ζῶσαν, as it reads in I, 30, ψυχὴν ζωῆς. Other instances from the Book of Genesis could be cited of the wide significance given therein to the expression which corresponds to "soul."

[181] *Domi.* Compare Aristotle: On the Generation of Animals, 736a, 24 to 737b, 7.

[182] Harvey: On Generation, LXXI, Syd. 511, l. 1–24; Op. Omn. 532, l. 9–29.

[183] *Neque sanguinis vim, virtutem, rationem, motum, aut calorem, ut cordis domum, habet.* Harvey: Exercise to Riolanus, II, Syd. 137, l. 16–17; Op. Omn. 137, l. 8–9.

[184] Hippocrates: On the Nature of Man, Lit. Vol. VI, 44, l. 7–10.

[185] Harvey: On Generation, XVII, Syd. 239, l. 13–23 and l. 29–31; Op. Omn. 253, l. 3–11 and l. 15–18.

[186] Harvey: On Generation, LVII, Syd. 430, l. 23–33; Op. Omn. 449, l. 11–21.

[187] *Promanat.*

[188] Harvey: On Generation, XLVII, Syd. 347, l. 26 to 348, l. 3; Op. Omn. 363, l. 18 to 364, l. 2.

[189] *Primigenia.*

[190] Harvey: On Generation, LI, Syd. 375, l. 40 to 376, l. 8; Op. Omn. 392, l. 3–10.

[191] Leviticus XVII, 11 and 14 — Harvey's own reference. Not these two verses merely, but the whole of chapter XVII, should be read, not only in the Authorized Version, but in the Revised Version also.

[192] Harvey: On Generation, LI, Syd. 376, l. 19–21; Op. Omn. 392, l. 20–22.

[193] Harvey: On Generation, LI, Syd. 377, l. 3–11; Op. Omn. 393, l. 7–14.

[194] Harvey: On Generation, LII, Syd. 380, l. 14–16; Op. Omn. 396, l. 18–20.

[195] Harvey: On Generation, LII, Syd. 381, l. 26–35; Op. Omn. 398, l. 1–8.

[196] Harvey: On Generation, LII, Syd. 391, l. 11–30; Op. Omn. 408, l. 8–22.

[197] Aristotle: On Soul, Book I, chapter 2 — Harvey's own reference. For Thales, Diogenes, Heraclitus, Alcmæon, and their

views, see also Zeller, Die Philosophie der Griechen, I Theeil, 5 Auflage, Leipsic, 1892.   For Critias, see William Smith, Dîictionary of Greek and Roman Biography and Mythology, Vol. I, London, 1880, 892.

²⁹⁸ Aristotle: History of Animals, I, chapter 19 — Harvey's ovwn reference. This should read III, chapter 19, 520b, 14–17 and 521la, 6–9.   The reference to Book I is an error of the press which has beeen copied without correction from the *Editio Princeps* in both tlhe Opera Omnia and the Sydenham translation. Aristotle: On tlhe Parts of Animals, II, chapter 3 (Harvey's own reference), 650b, 2—8.

²⁹⁹ Harvey: On Generation, LII, Syd. 380, l. 37 to 381, l. 2ε0; Op. Omn. 397, l. 8–27.

³⁰⁰ Plato: Phædo, 96b: Platonis Dialogi, Hermann-Wohlraιb, Vol. I, 142, l. 2–3.

³⁰¹ Censorinus: De Die Natali, chapter VI, § 1, Edition Hultscːh, 1867, 10.

³⁰² Empedocles: Fragment 105, l. 3; Diels, Poetarum Philosιophorum Fragmenta, Berlin, 1901, 146, constituting Vol. III of Wilamowitz-Moellendorf, Poetarum Græcorum Fragmenta. Seee also Zeller, Die Philosophie der Griechen, I Theil, 5 Auflage, 189ι2.

³⁰³ Theophrastus: Opera Omnia: On Sensation and Sensibιle Things, II, (10), Edition Wimmer, 323a, Paris, Didot, 1866.

³⁰⁴ Compare Aristotle: On Soul, 404b, 27–30.

³⁰⁵ Aristotle: History of Animals, 520b, 14–17.

³⁰⁶ Harvey: On Generation, LII, Syd. 382, l. 18–21; Op. Omn. 398, l. 24–27.

³⁰⁷ Harvey: On Generation, LII, Syd. 380, l. 3–6; Op. Omn. 396, l. 9–12.

³⁰⁸ Harvey: On Generation, LII, Syd. 390, l. 35 to 391, l. 2; Op. Omn. 407, l. 25–30.

³⁰⁹ See Harvey: Letter to Hofmann, Syd. 595, l. 6–15; Op. Omn. 635, l. 10–17.

³¹⁰ See J. B. Meyer: Aristoteles' Thierkunde, 1855, 411, l. 14 tto 413, l. 2.

³¹¹ *Calor animalis.*

³¹² Harvey: On Generation, LXXI, Syd. 501, l. 29 to 502, l. 16 and 502, l. 38 to 503, l. 20; Op. Omn. 523, l. 1–16 and 524, l. 8–24.

³¹³ Harvey: On Generation, LXXI, Syd. 504, l. 6–10; Op. Omn. 525, l. 13–16.

³¹⁴ Harvey: On Generation, LXXI, Syd. 504, l. 16–34; Op. Omn. 525, l. 20 to 526, l. 2.

[315] Aristotle: On the Generation of Animals, Book II, chapter 3 (Harvey's own reference), 736*b*, 29–31.

[316] The Latin translation of this passage which is quoted by Harvey reads: "*Omnis animae sive potentia*, etc." The Greek text of Aristotle reads: "πάσης μὲν οὖν ψυχῆς δύναμις," κ.τ.λ., meaning "the faculty of every soul." In the part of the chapter which just precedes this passage Aristotle discourses of "the nutritive soul," "the sensory soul," and "the intellectual soul"; and the context makes it clear that the words of the passage quoted by Harvey refer to the faculty of every kind of soul, and not simply to the faculty of the soul of every living being.

[317] ἑτέρου σώματος ἔοικε κεκοινωνηκέναι, κ.τ.λ. The Latin translation of these words, which is quoted by Harvey, reads: "*corpus aliud participare videtur*." Regarding the significance of κεκοινωνηκέναι in this passage compare Aristotle: Economics, 1343*a*, 10–12; although this treatise is now believed to be not by Aristotle himself, but by a later member of his school.

[318] Aristotle: On the Generation of Animals, 736*b*, 33 to 737*a*, 1.

[319] πνεῦμα (*Pneuma*).

[320] The following are the words of Aristotle which Harvey omits from his quotation:—

"and, moreover, as the souls differ one from another in nobility and ignobleness, so too does the nature aforesaid differ." (Aristotle: On the Generation of Animals, 736*b*, 31–33.)

If these words be read in their proper connection, it becomes clear that "the nature which is analogous to the element of the stars" is the same as "the nature aforesaid" (ἡ τοιαύτη φύσις), which is the "body other than the so-called elements and more divine." Fire is repeatedly styled a "body" by Aristotle, it being one of the four "simple bodies" (ἁπλᾶ σώματα) or elements. Compare Aristotle: On Generation and Corruption, 330*b*, 1–3. We shall find that Harvey in his turn styles fire a "body" (*corpus*). See Harvey: On Generation, LXXI, Syd. 506, l. 26–31; Op. Omn. 527, l. 28 to 528, l. 1.

The Latin translation of Aristotle which Harvey quotes reads, in dealing with the "spirits": "*spiritus qui in semine spumosoque corpore continetur, et natura quae in eo spiritu est proportione respondens elemento stellarum*." (Aristotle: On the Generation of Animals, Vol. III, 360*b*, 4–5.) The Greek text reads: τὸ ἐμπεριλαμβανόμενον ἐν τῷ σπέρματι καὶ ἐν τῷ ἀφρώδει πνεῦμα καὶ ἡ ἐν τῷ πνεύματι φύσις, ἀνάλογον οὖσα τῷ τῶν ἄστρων στοιχείῳ (736b, 35 to 737a, 1). Two manuscripts omit "ἐν" before "τῷ πνεύματι."

In the chapter immediately preceding Aristotle says: —

"Not only does a liquid become thick which is made of water and earthy matter, but also one made of water and spirits; even as foam thickens and whitens; and the smaller and less conspicuous the bubbles are, the whiter and stiffer does the mass appear. Oil, too, is affected in the same way; for it becomes thick when mixed with spirits, so that, as it whitens, it thickens; what is watery within it being separated by the heat, and becoming spirits. . . . For the reasons aforesaid the semen, too, is stiff and white as it issues from within, since it contains much hot spirits due to the interior heat. But after the exit of the semen, when its heat has exhaled and its air has cooled, it liquefies and darkens. For in drying semen, as in phlegm, the water remains and perhaps some little earthy matter. The semen then is a combination of spirits and water, the spirits being hot air; so the semen, being derived from water, is naturally liquid. . . . The cause of the whiteness of the semen is that the generative medium (ἡ γονή) is foam, and that foam is white. . . . It seems not to have escaped even the ancients that the nature of semen is foamy; at all events they named from this property (δυνάμεως) the goddess who rules coition." (Aristotle: On the Generation of Animals, 735b, 8–16; 735b, 32 to 736a, 2; 736a, 13–14 and a, 18–21.)

A very ancient poem, ascribed to Hesiod, relates the myth of Aphrodite and says that she was so called by gods and men "because she was produced in foam." (Theogony, l. 197–198.) The "air" [ἀήρ] of one of the foregoing passages from Aristotle is of course not atmospheric air, but something aëriform produced by heat, as the context shows. In the same treatise he speaks of the presence, within the early embryo which has never breathed, of spirits (πνεῦμα) due to heat and moisture, "the one active, the other passive." (On the Generation of Animals, 741b, 37 to 742a, 16.)

[111] The Latin translation quoted by Harvey renders the Greek words "οὐδὲ φαίνεται συνιστάμενον πυρουμένοις οὔτ' [ἐν] ὑγροῖς οὔτ' ἐν ξηροῖς οὐθέν". (737a, 1–3) by the misleading words "neque constitui quidquam densis vel humidis vel siccis videntur." Therefore, in translating this passage into English, it has seemed necessary to make it intelligible by giving to the word "πυρουμένοις" its proper meaning, rather than by rendering literally the earlier translator's ill-chosen Latin word "densis."

[112] The Latin quoted by Harvey, viz.: "qui semine continetur," scarcely gives the force of the original Greek "ἡ διὰ τοῦ σπέρματος."

(737a, 3–4), which Greek words, rather than the Latin, are rendered in the present English translation.

[323] ἀλλὰ κἄν τι περίττωμα τύχῃ τῆς φύσεως ὂν ἕτερον. κ. τ. λ. (737a, 4–5). Compare the construction of this passage with that of the following: διὰ τὸ πλησιαίτερα ἡμῶν εἶναι καὶ τῆς φύσεως οἰκειότερα. κ.τ.λ. Aristotle: On the Parts of Animals, 645a, 2–3.

[324] Aristotle: On the Generation of Animals, 736b, 33 to 737a, 7. In translating into English the foregoing Aristotelian passages the present writer has sought rather to indicate than to smooth away the ruggedness of the original Greek. Harvey quotes these passages verbatim from a Latin translation which may be found in Volume III of the Berlin Academy's quarto edition of Aristotle's works. This translation was made in the fifteenth century by Theodore Gaza, a learned Greek of Thessalonica, who had fled from the conquering Turks to Italy, where he learned Latin not long before his thirtieth year. Gaza was neither physician nor biologist. In view of these facts we need not wonder that his Latin version of Aristotle On the Generation of Animals is occasionally unsatisfactory, as we have seen. In the edition of the Greek text of Aristotle's History of Animals, published by Teubner in 1907 (Aristotelis De Animalibus Historia, textum recognovit Leonardus Dittmeyer, 1907, Leipsic, p. XXII, l. 1–5), the editor says in his Latin preface, regarding Gaza's Latin Translation of the History of Animals: "There is need of caution, if we wish to unearth the Greek text from his interpretation."

[325] *Respondens*, not *proportione respondens.*

[326] Harvey: On Generation, LXXI, Syd. 505, l. 18 to 506, l. 16; Op. Omn. 526, l. 20 to 527, l. 20.

[327] Harvey: On Generation, LXXI, Syd. 508, l. 22–38; Op. Omn. 529, l. 24 to 530, l. 5.

[328] The sources, contained in Aristotle's own works, of the foregoing brief sketch of his conception of the universe, are as follows: On Heaven, the whole of the treatise; On Generation and Corruption, the whole of the treatise; Physics, Book IV, chapter 14, 223b, 15 to 224a, 2; Meteorology, Book I, chapters 1, 2, 3, and 9; Metaphysics, Book XI, chapter 7, 1072b, 28–30, and chapter 8; Nicomachean Ethics, Book VI, chapter 7, 1141a, 33 to b, 2; On the Parts of Animals, Book I, chapters 4 and 5, 644b, 20–25; Book II, chapter 10, 656a, 3–8; On the Generation of Animals, Book IV, chapter 10. The treatise entitled "On the Universe: To Alexander," is not a genuine work of Aristotle. See V. Rose: De Aristotelis

Librorum Ordine et Auctoritate, 90–100. Besides the foregoing Aristotelian texts, see Prantl's note, number 37, on pages 303–307 of his edition of Aristotle's treatise On Heaven and On Generation and Corruption, and the references to other writers contained in the said note.

[329] Aristotle: On Heaven, 269a, 5–7.

[330] Aristotle: Meteorology, 339b, 25–26.

[331] Aristotle: On Heaven, 269a, 30–32.

[332] Aristotle: On Heaven, 269b, 15–17.

[333] Aristotle: On Heaven, 270b, 1–5 and 20–24. Aristotle accepts the derivation of αἰθέρα from ἀεὶ θεῖν. Modern philology rejects this.

[334] Aristotle: Meteorology, 339b, 17–19.

[335] Aristotle: On Heaven, 289a, 13–16.

[336] Milton: Paradise Lost, III, l. 716–721.

[337] See pp. 119–121.

[338] Aristotle: Physics, 194b, 13.

[339] Aristotle: On the Generation of Animals, 731b, 35 to 732a, 1. This is a small part of a passage of which the whole should be read, viz.: 731b, 24 to 732a, 6. Compare On Generation and Corruption, 337a, 34 to 338b, 19.

[340] Aristotle: History of Animals, 511b, 1–4.

[341] Aristotle: On the Parts of Animals, 652b, 23–26. On the Generation of Animals, 742b, 35 to 743a, 1.

[342] Compare Aristotle: On the Parts of Animals, 645a, 26 to 645b, 14.

[343] Aristotle: On the Generation of Animals, Book II, chapter 3 — Harvey's own reference.

[344] Harvey: On Generation, XXVIII, Syd. 285, l. 22–36; Op. Omn. 300, l. 9–21.

[345] Compare Harvey: On Generation, LXXI, Syd. 502, l. 25–37; Op. Omn. 523, l. 24 to 524, l. 7.

[346] E.g. Harvey: On Generation, LXXI, Syd. 507, l. 32–36; Op. Omn. 529, l. 2–5.

[347] See pp. 119–121.

[348] Cicero et al.

[349] See Aristotle: On Heaven, 269b, 18 to 270a, 12. Compare J. B. Meyer: Aristoteles' Thierkunde, II Abschnitt, § 2, 407, l. 20 to 413, l. 27.

[350] Aristotle: On the Parts of Animals, 645a, 26 to b, 14; especially 645b, 6–10. See also Poetics, 1457b, 16–19.

[351] See p. 120.

[352] See pp. 119–121.

[353] See p. 120.

[354] Harvey: On Generation, LXXI, Syd. 507, l. 37 to 508, l. 13; Op. Omn. 529, l. 6–16.

[355] Harvey: On Generation, LXXII, Syd. 513, l. 1–24 and 516, l. 14–17; Op. Omn. 534, l. 12 to 535, l. 6 and 537, l. 26–28.

[356] Harvey: On Generation, LXXII, Syd. 517, l. 19–22; Op. Omn. 539, l. 3–5. For the views of Empedocles and Democritus, see Zeller: Philosophie der Griechen, I Theil, 2 Hälfte, 5 Auflage, 750–777 and 837–898. For the views of the chemists, see Roscoe and Schorlemmer: A Treatise on Chemistry, Vol. I, 1878, 3–11.

[357] Harvey: On Generation, LXXII, Syd. 517, l. 27–32; Op. Omn. 539, l. 9–14. The words at the end of the quotation read, in Harvey's text: "*aut principia esse corporum similarium.*" The "*corpora similaria*" or "*partes similares*" are the ὁμοιομερῆ of Aristotle, which in anatomy answer, nearly, to the "tissues" of modern parlance. See Aristotle: On the Parts of Animals, 646a, 12–24.

[358] See p. 105.

[359] See p. 116.

[360] See p. 117.

[361] See pp. 119–121 and notes 321–324.

[362] Harvey: On Generation, LXXI, Syd. 507, l. 32–36; Op. Omn. 529, l. 2–5.

[363] *Sanguinis calor est animalis, quatenus scilicet in operationibus suis ab anima gubernatur;* etc.

[364] Harvey: On Generation, LXXI, Syd. 508, l. 14–17; Op. Omn. 529, l. 17–20.

[365] Compare Aristotle: Meteorology, 339a, 11–32.

[366] κόσμος means both "order" and "ornament."

[367] Harvey: On Generation, LXXI, Syd. 508, l. 22–29; Op. Omn. 529, l. 24–30.

[368] Compare Aristotle: On the Generation of Animals, 737a, 16 to b, 7, especially a, 30–34; 741a, 3–32; 750b, 3–26; 757b, 14–19, and b, 23–27.

[369] Harvey: On Generation, LII, Syd. 381, l. 20–25; Op. Omn. 397, l. 27–30. Compare the same, LIV, Syd. 402, l. 10–27; Op. Omn. 419, l. 23 to 420, l. 8.

[370] See p. 121.

[371] *Fateatur.*

[372] Harvey: On Generation, XLVII, Syd. 350, l. 2–16; Op. Omn. 365, l. 31 to 366, l. 11.

[173] See pp. 122–123.

[174] See p. 119. See also Aristotle: On the Generation of Animals, 736b, 30.

[175] Harvey: On Generation, LXXI, Syd. 506, l. 26–29; Op. Omn. 527, l. 28–31. Compare Aristotle: On Generation and Corruption, 330b, 1–3, and elsewhere.

[176] Harvey: On Generation, LXXI, Syd. 506, l. 17 to 507, l. 15; Op. Omn. 527, l. 21 to 528, l. 20. Do., Syd. 508, l. 30 to 509, l. 24; Op. Omn. 530, l. 5–27.

[177] Harvey: On Generation, LXXI, Syd. 506, l. 29–30; Op. Omn. 527, l. 32.

[178] *Participare.*

[179] Harvey: On Generation, LXXI, Syd. 507, l. 6–15; Op. Omn. 528, l. 13–20.

[180] Aristotle: On the Generation of Animals, 736a, 24 to 737b, 7. Gaza's Latin translation of this chapter may be found on page 350 of the third volume of the Prussian Academy's edition of Aristotle's Works.

[181] Compare p. 120.

[182] Aristotle: Meteorology, 382a, 6–7.

[183] Aristotle: Meteorology, 340b, 22–23.

[184] Harvey: On Generation, LXXII, Syd. 518, l. 15–36; Op. Omn. 540, l. 1–17.

[185] Harvey: Prelectiones, 98 left.

[186] Cicero: On the Nature of the Gods, Mül. 60, l. 23 to 61, l. 2.

[187] Aristotle: On Youth and Old Age and on Life and Death, 469b, 15–16.

[188] Aristotle: On Respiration, 474a, 26–28.

[189] συναίτιον.

[190] τῶν δὲ φύσει συνισταμένων πάντων.

[191] λόγος.

[192] Aristotle: On Soul, 416a, 9–18.

[193] See pp. 119 and 140.

[194] Compare Aristotle: History of Animals, 539a, 15–25; 550b, 30 to 551a, 13: On the Generation of Animals, 761a, 12 to 763b, 16.

[195] κινοῦσα.

[196] Aristotle: Meteorology, 364b, 20–23.

[197] κινοῦντα.

[198] Aristotle: Metaphysics, 1071a, 11–17. Compare Physics, 194b, 29–32 and On the Generation of Animals, 716a, 4–7.

³⁹⁹ τὸ δημιουργοῦν. Aristotle: On the Generation of Animals, 738b, 20–21.

⁴⁰⁰ Aristotle: On the Generation of Animals, 762b, 2–4.

⁴⁰¹ Aristotle: On the Generation of Animals, 738b, 25–26. Compare 716a, 4–7.

⁴⁰² Aristotle: On Respiration, 479a, 29–30.

⁴⁰³ Aristotle: On the Generation of Animals, 741a, 3–32, 757b, 14–27.

⁴⁰⁴ Aristotle: On the Generation of Animals, 716a, 13–17.

⁴⁰⁵ Strictly speaking, it is left uncertain by the Greek text whether the verb translated by the words "when . . . inclusion . . . has taken place" refers to "heat," or to "soul," or to both. This uncertainty, however, does not affect the sense, as both the expression "psychical heat," and the words which follow it, imply the association of heat and soul with one another. A line or two beyond this quoted passage, Aristotle speaks of "the inclusion of the psychical principle."

⁴⁰⁶ Owing to the vagueness of the word συνίσταται this must be translated here by a periphrasis such as "an individual is formed." The verb συνιστάναι is used by Aristotle to express not only the immediate result of spontaneous generation, or the production of the embryo in sexual generation, but also the curdling of milk, the condensation of vapor into water, and even the constitution of the universe.

⁴⁰⁷ θερμαινομένων τῶν σωματικῶν ὑγρῶν.

⁴⁰⁸ Aristotle: On the Generation of Animals, 762a, 18–24.

⁴⁰⁹ ἡ δὲ θάλαττα . . . σωματώδης, πολλῷ μᾶλλον τοῦ ποτίμου . . . ἐστί. Aristotle: On the Generation of Animals, 761b, 8–12. Compare 761a, 33 to b, 2.

⁴¹⁰ περίττωμα.

⁴¹¹ I.e., the female animal.

⁴¹² I.e., in the higher animals.

⁴¹³ συνίστησιν.

⁴¹⁴ κίνησιν ἐντίθησιν.

⁴¹⁵ Aristotle: On the Generation of Animals, 762a, 35 to b, 19.

⁴¹⁶ Aristotle: On the Generation of Animals, 729a, 34 to b, 21; and the passages cited on p. 145.

⁴¹⁷ Compare Aristotle: On the Generation of Animals, 743a, 26 to b, 5.

⁴¹⁸ φρόνησις. Hippocrates: On the Sacred Disease, Lit. Vol. VI, 390, l. 10 to 394, l. 8.

⁴¹⁹ Genesis: II, 7.

[420] Aristotle: On Soul, 410b, 27 to 411a, 2.

[421] Aristotle: On the Generation of Animals, 736a, 22 to 737b, 7.

[422] Aristotle: On Soul, 410b, 16 to 411a, 22.

[423] Aristotle: On the Generation of Animals, 728b, 21–32.

[424] Aristotle: On the Generation of Animals, 728a, 9–11.

[425] Aristotle: On the Generation of Animals, 763a, 24 to b, 4.

[426] Aristotle: On the Generation of Animals, 736b, 35–37. Gaza translates the foregoing as follows: *spiritus qui in semine spumosoque corpore continetur.* Aristotle: Op. Ed. Acad. Reg. Boruss. Vol. III, 360b, l. 4.

[427] Hesiod: Theogony, l. 188–200. Compare Aristotle: On the Generation of Animals, 736a, 18–21, and see note 320. The same myth is referred to by Harvey in his turn: On Generation, L, Syd. 368, l. 1–7; Op. Omn. 383, l. 18–22.

[428] Aristotle: On Heaven, 289a, 11–19. The derivation now accepted of the word "ether," αἰθήρ, is from αἴθω, "I kindle"; which substantiates Aristotle's account of the view which he combats. Indeed, Aristotle himself says: "Anaxagoras, however, has not employed this word correctly; for he uses the word 'ether' in place of 'fire.'" On Heaven, 270b, 24–25.

[429] The ether.

[430] Aristotle: On Heaven, 289a, 19–22 and 26–35.

[431] Aristotle: Meteorology, 341a, 35–36.

[432] See pp. 119 and 140.

[433] Harvey: On Generation, L, Syd. 368, l. 12–25; Op. Omn. 383, l. 26 to 384, l. 4.

[434] *Quod sponte nascentibus fæcunditatem affert.*

[435] Harvey: On Generation, L, Syd. 370, l. 27–34; Op. Omn. 386, l. 14–20. See note 439.

[436] *In sponte nascentibus vermis.*

[437] *Conclusae humiditatis.*

[438] Harvey: On Generation, LVI, Syd. 414, l. 32 to 415, l. 9; Op. Omn. 433, l. 5–11.

[439] Compare Aristotle: History of Animals, 539b, 17–25. Harvey: On the Motion, etc., XVII, Syd. 75, l. 23–29; Op. Omn. 77, l. 1–6. Harvey: On Generation, I, Syd. 170, l. 32–36; Op. Omn. 182, l. 20–23; Do. L, Syd. 367, l. 30–36; Op. Omn. 383, l. 10–15; Do. LXII, Syd. 457, l. 18–27; Op. Omn. 477, l. 4–12. Harvey: On Parturition, Syd. 524, l. 31–39; Op. Omn. 544, l. 13–19. T. H. Huxley: Encyclopædia Britannica, 9th ed., Vol. VIII, Article on "Evolution," 746, especially 746a, 43 to b, 2. W. K. Brooks:

William Harvey as an Embryologist, Johns Hopkins Hospital Bulletin, Vol. VIII, 1897, 169a, 7 to 170b, 26.

[440] Compare Aristotle: On the Generation of Animals, 724a, 14 to 727b, 33.

[441] Harvey: On Generation, LII, Syd. 381, l. 36 to 383, l. 7; Op. Omn. 398, l. 9–16.

[442] *Intellectu.*

[443] *Ratiocinio.*

[444] Harvey: On Generation, LXXI, Syd. 507, l. 16–26; Op. Omn. 528, l. 21–29.

[445] Aristotle: Meteorology, 339a, 21–24.

[446] Aristotle: Physics, 223b, 24–26.

[447] Milton: Paradise Lost, Book VIII, l. 15–178.

[448] Harvey: Exercise to Riolanus, II, Syd. 132, l. 9–11; Op. Omn. 132, l. 2–3.

[449] Harvey: Exercise to Riolanus, II, Syd. 123, l. 21–33; Op. Omn. 123, l. 15–17.

[450] *Aërem;* i.e., aëriform vapor.

[451] Compare Aristotle: On Sleep and Waking, 457b, 29 to 458a, 5.

[452] Harvey: On the Motion, etc., VIII, Syd. 46, l. 25–33; Op. Omn. 48, l. 28 to 49, l. 2.

[453] *Quatenus est elementaris.*

[454] The goddess of the domestic fire.

[455] Compare Plato: Timæus, 48e to 50a; 54c to 62c, and 76c to 80d; Plato: Philebus, 28e to 30a.

[456] Harvey: On Generation, LXXI, Syd. 510, l. 5–40; Op. Omn. 531, l. 12 to 532, l. 9.

[457] Æschylus: Agamemnon, l. 5–6.

INDEX

191

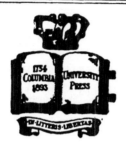